NURSE EDUCATION AND THE CURRICULUM

Nurse Education and the Curriculum

A Curricular Model

Fred Greaves, SRN, DN, RNT, Dip.Ad.Ed., MEd.

Advanced Nursing and Health Studies Unit,
Liverpool Polytechnic

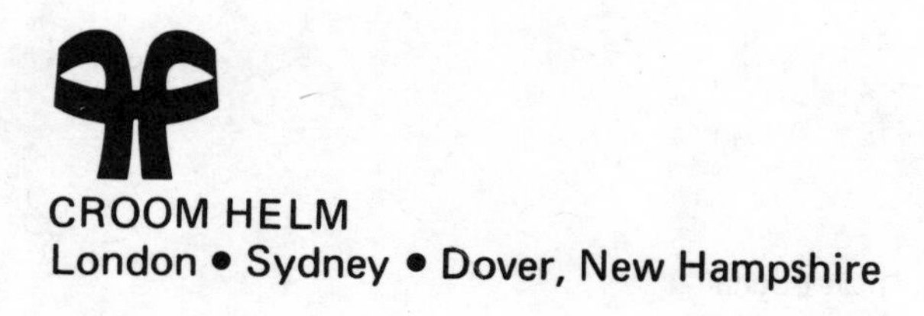
CROOM HELM
London • Sydney • Dover, New Hampshire

Croom Helm Ltd, Provident House, Burrell Row,
Beckenham, Kent BR3 1AT
Croom Helm Australia Pty Ltd, Suite 4, 6th Floor,
64-76 Kippax Street, Surry Hills, NSW 2010, Australia
Croom Helm, 51 Washington Street,
Dover, New Hampshire 03820, USA
Reprinted 1985

British Library Cataloguing in Publication Data

Greaves, Fred
Nurse education and the curriculum.
1. Nursing – Study and teaching
2. Curriculum planning
I. Title
610.73'07'11 RT73

ISBN 0-7099-1179-3 Pbk

Printed and bound in Great Britain
by Billing & Sons Limited, Worcester.

CONTENTS

LIST OF FIGURES AND TABLES

Figures

Tables

To Rosemary, a dedicated nurse and gifted teacher

PREFACE

The nursing process, the curriculum process and theoretical nursing models are essential areas of concern for those nurses who are involved with the design, planning and implementation of nurse educational programmes. This book attempts to review and bring together appropriate elements of these three important areas of knowledge. A critical analysis of nursing theory and of the relationship of theory to practice, and an overview of nursing models is presented along with an examination of general curriculum theory and practice, and possible nursing curriculum applications. Antecedent and specific nursing knowledge is conceptually identified and differentiated for potential curricular applications.

In the final chapter the author presents his personal view of a nursing curriculum model which is suggested as a guiding conceptual framework for curriculum thought and planning. The model specifies complementary frames of reference that bring together the curriculum process, the nursing process and elements of nursing models that are viewed as significant for the education of nurses.

The book does not set out to give detailed prepared examples of curricular content and materials, but attempts in a modest way to provoke and stimulate curriculum thinking about the conceptual areas and issues presented.

It is hoped that the material presented will be of use to all professional nurses who are concerned with the educational preparation of nurses at whatever level that preparation might be. This would include nurse teachers, clinical nurse teachers, nurse education managers and practising nurses with an input to basic nurse preparation and to continuing nurse education. Student nurse teachers, student clinical teachers, student teachers of health visiting and midwifery, and intending teachers in the paramedical professions may also find the content relevant to their future educational role.

Post-registration nurses and postgraduate nurses attending diploma, first degree or higher degree courses in which there is a professional nursing component with a curriculum perspective should also find the book a useful supplement and guide to their reading.

1 NURSING THEORY AND PRACTICE: A CURRICULAR DILEMMA

(i) Introduction

A theoretical framework for the practice of nursing is slowly developing and with it the very nature of nursing itself is being gradually identified. Yet, at the same time the traditional practices of past generations of nurses are fundamentally unchanged and can be seen as normative practices in most countries today. Consequently, there exists a pressing need to identify and agree which theoretical and practical aspects of nursing are those which will operate in such a way that adequate standards are achieved. These need to be based in objective thinking and capable of meeting the health care requirements of modern society.

Nursing and nurses are still faced with problems of their public and professional image. This can be seen in attempts to move from a position of semi-professional to one of full professional status, a shift which inevitably raises questions of role identification and occupational accountability. Both the nursing service and nursing education are still seen to be seeking a better way to prepare future nurse practitioners in a more rational way within health service organisational contexts which are constantly changing.

These are the most significant of the major issues facing nurses in many countries today. They are not necessarily seen as new problems, for they have been recognised for some time, but they are problems which are significant in any projection for the development of future nursing curricula. Any curriculum designed for nursing must represent the present realities of the world of nursing and take account of major problems and issues. It is increasingly recognised that the educational arrangements for the training of nurses are inadequate for today's health care requirements. Public expectations have increased on the question of quality of care and the delivery of nursing can no longer be based on a medical model. Just as health is no longer the absence of disease, health care is no longer defined as the provision of medical diagnosis and treatment. For nurses this means that the caring aspect of nursing has to be more accurately defined and described and must include a greater emphasis on health teaching, health maintenance, the prevention of illness and caring ways of reducing human suffering. A basic examination of the field of nursing reveals great diversity in what counts as the practice of nursing. The concept of nursing in the past has been too simplistic and the caring element, the 'core' mechanisms of nursing (the carative factors) have to be viewed in the context of a science of care. This means that nursing has to identify and develop its own body of knowledge and emerge as a scientific discipline with its practice base derived from scientific knowledge and research.

The development of a curriculum in the United Kingdom for nursing education is changing in response to changing nursing practices. The theoretical underpinnings of education are increasingly derived from data collected by practitioners engaged in ongoing research in nursing practice settings. Consequently new ideas, exploration, experimentation and innovation must be the focus of nursing education.

Previously in the United Kingdom no real use has been made of curriculum theory and practice and there has been little in the way of objective thinking in curriculum terms; the advantages of using curricula processes has only recently been recognised. The current schemes for training nurses at the pre-registration level (up to state registration) are intensively being revised and re-thought and a complete revision is currently underway. The previous educational arrangements have been seen as inadequate for the changing circumstances of today.

In this book three major perspectives will be attempted which will culminate in a proposed curriculum model for nursing theory and practice.

(1) A new emerging theoretical focus in nursing will be retrospectively viewed and an analysis made of the current representations of nursing knowledge. This focus will relate to the major issues and problems associated with theory and practice. It will also take into account conceptualisations of nursing, frames of reference for nursing theory, and a critical review of nursing models.

(2) An examination of general curriculum theory and its relevance for nursing, and suggested adaptations which can be used for the design of a nursing curriculum, will be made.

(3) An attempt will be made to present an outline model for the nursing curriculum which will take account of general curriculum theory and relate to current educational problems in professional nursing. Although the main direction of the study is towards problems associated with curriculum content,

intentions, planning and evaluation and the curricular processes concerned with these, the issues involved will raise questions of a philosophical nature related to theory and practice, and questions of a psychological nature concerned with learning and clinical nursing pedagogy.

Professions longer established than nursing have usually based their educational arrangements on clearly identified goals, and tend to have an objective view of things such as scope, content and method, within their training and educational practices. As nursing is still attempting to identify its unique functions and purposes the consequent intentions for education are unclear. Retrospectively the 1950s can be seen as years that saw the beginning of the search for the nature of nursing and its own particular form of objectivity, a feature characteristic of any academic or professional discipline. The 1960s saw a sharpening of this focus directed at nursing theory and also a delineation of nursing activity into role and administrative emphasis. This shift reflected the attempts of nurses to evolve a clearer professional identity. Yet perhaps the most significant events of the 1960s were the exploration and attempts to develop early forms of nursing theory. Many nursing models were produced and the profession could be clearly seen to move in two major directions: first, the seeking of professional identity, and secondly, the securing of a body of knowledge sound enough to underpin professional nursing practice. Both directions were clearly dependent on systematising both nursing practice and nursing research.

The 1970s and the early 1980s have seen a continuous and increasing emphasis on all these fronts with general concern directed towards developing some agreement about such important issues as professional and role identity, the general development of professional nursing education and the organisation of a knowledge base for nursing practice. Rationalisation of effort, and systematic and economic approaches were increasingly seen to be *a priori* for a systematic development of nursing knowledge, much of which would be derived from research.

(ii) Nursing Theory and Practice: A Dilemma for the Curriculum

In the development of a curriculum for nursing there is quite clearly a need for the relationship of theory and practice to be seen as equally important, interrelated and integrated into the very idea of nursing.

Because nursing is a 'practical activity' often undertaken by semi-trained or untrained people, theoretical assumptions about nursing are often regarded with suspicion, or often associated with such terms as 'woolly mindedness' or 'impractical'. Consequently it has often been believed that there can be no real nursing theories because all the relevant theory applied in nursing is borrowed from other disciplines. If this is the case, if nursing has no unique function, so the argument goes, there is no reason for the professional education of nurses. This form of argument rests on an artificial distinction that attempts to divorce theory from practice. The idea that nursing is practical and, therefore, not theoretical shows an inadequate understanding of the interrelationship of theory and practice.

It would be illogical to suggest that there could be a single 'theory of nursing' but there can be theories about nursing in the sense that one can be involved in theorising about what it is to be a nurse or what the job of nursing involves nurses in. There can also be theorising within nursing in the sense that biological and behavioural knowledge can support a particular nursing action in a nurse-patient interaction. Clearly both forms of theorising stand in close relationship to practice and necessary justifications for their inclusion in a nursing curriculum could no doubt be made. However a necessary distinction would need to be made between the two in terms of selection in relationship to the nursing content of a curriculum.

In viewing nursing as an area of knowledge for the curriculum there can be no useful purpose gained by creating a dichotomy between theory and practice. Such a division would be artificial, for all practical activities are preceded by thought, guided by thought, and however simplistic must be taking account of theory. Knowing what to do and how to do it is inextricably bound up with the performance itself and knowing and doing belong to the same locus of existence and the same order of awareness. In the final analysis, knowledge cannot realistically be called either practical or theoretical and for curricula purposes nursing content must be concerned with describing, explaining and controlling the phenomena of nursing patients. Any initial discrimination of subject matter into practice and theory when seeking purposeful curriculum organisation is inevitably bound to increase already existing artificial divisions. Knowledge in nursing cannot usefully be viewed primarily for its own sake or valued for its own sake because in this way knowledge is seen purely as theory and sterile theory at that. Knowledge in nursing must be viewed as arising from problematic situations (realities) and directed toward the settlement of present and future problems. Consequently no sharp distinction should be made between the theoretical and the practical.

The theory/practice dichotomy has led nurses to direct their attention to nursing theory and its possible relationship with nursing practice. The process of nursing itself is also receiving considerable attention and the conceptual underpinning of nursing theory and attempts at securing a 'core theory' of nursing have occupied the attention of nursing academics and practitioners over the last decade. At the same time nurses are also beginning to respond more positively to patterns of change which are seen to be influencing a re-shaping of nursing practice, a re-evaluation of traditional roles, a re-identification of standards of patient care, and a review of the educational preparation of nursing practitioners. As nursing practice emerges from a culture tradition deeply rooted in the past into its current transitionary stage, a new scientific foundation is being sought as the base for modern professional nursing. Subsequently, attempts to establish nursing as a recognised profession are reflected in the pursuit of a distinctive body of knowledge which rests on objectivity, rationality, unification and a reconstruction of nursing, whereby a realistic set of applications can be made through nursing practice, nursing research and nursing education.

The assumption that nursing is a purely practical activity and not a theoretical one is still held by less enlightened nurses. Yet it is exceedingly difficult to provide effective and good quality nursing care without certain theoretical applications within nursing. A major requirement in nursing today is the need to make more effective use of concepts in order to reach agreed conceptualisations of the nature of nursing.

(iii) Concepts, Theories and Knowledge

Inquiry, or directed thinking, has its origin in a conceptual structure. *Concepts* themselves are products of a person observing instances (e.g. nursing) about real world phenomena or realities. They may be described as extensions of percepts (things perceived), as a grasp of overall structure obtained by the isolation and identification of relevant factors and relationships. Conceptualisations about nursing enable complex phenomena observed in nursing situations to be modelled as simplified approximations of the real world of nursing. In nursing activities, general concepts are necessary to guide the behaviour of nurses in caring for patients. Conceptualisations are also required of the essential structure of nursing so that practitioners, teachers and learners can respond effectively to the various types of nursing experience. The notion of a general concept of nursing is also well known among nurses to be crucial to any emerging knowledge base because a general concept will allow the identification of those elements upon which the nurse should focus to make inferences from the observed empirical data of nursing actions. It is also seen as a necessary guide to the design and production of a nursing care system such as the 'nursing process'.

In nursing contexts, conceptual analysis may help nurses to identify important aspects of the actual activity of nursing and provide a base for constructing theories that will be effective in nursing. By means of concepts and propositions built upon them, aspects are identified which are to be considered when attempting to represent those activities which we wish to call nursing. Using conceptual analysis an exposition of the nature of nursing can be reached through a process of building conceptual frameworks and eventually theories. By means of theory organisation ultimately a system of nursing knowledge is produced.

A *theory* is much more complex and is usually seen as a way of making sense of experience by looking at the relationships among particular events. Like concepts, theories are abstract and symbolic reconstructions of reality. Neither concepts nor theories strictly speaking describe the empirical world; concepts classify aspects of that world for the purposes of analytical description, while theories in nursing will provide explanations or reasons for the 'truth' of those descriptions. In this sense a theory or theories in nursing will ultimately represent a systematic frame of reference that can account for particular kinds of nursing events. To achieve such a logical and systematic collection of theories as a reference frame, nurses have to subject their theoretical formulations to empirical testing which may be derived by analytic induction or deductively from a set of premises.

The validity of a theory lies in its 'fit' to empirical events, and for nurses this means testing to explain, to account for and predict the empirical events within nursing contexts. In this way, theorising as a cognitive process in nursing will necessarily include both deductive and inductive elements and their application to what has been identified as nursing. The nature of nursing can be explained then in the light of our inductive *knowledge* and the empirical events of nursing activity and reconstructing that knowledge into a deductive system of testable propositions through a systematic analysis of evidence.

(iv) Current Theory in Nursing

During the last two decades (most notable in the United States of America) some progress has been made in an attempt to free nursing from practice and control of a so-called 'medical-model' and to conceptualise nursing as a practice-based profession in its own right. Significant within this intention is the search for nursing knowledge which is valid and recognisable both inside and outside the world of nursing. It is in this direction that the nursing theorists of the 1960s and 1970s attempted to unfold theories that were unique (or considered unique) to nursing and to evolve theoretical frameworks that also borrowed from established knowledge in other sciences, to guide nursing practice and research, and to assist in the development of nursing curricula.

In each instance the relationship between the developing nursing theories and nursing educational thinking has been problematic for curriculum developers and curriculum users. The central problem has been that there is no single neat, tidy, all generic set of theories that will adequately account for the present nursing practices and there are still nurses who feel that it is unlikely that there ever will be. Like in the teaching profession, one set of theories to provide for practice is not available or perhaps even desirable. Equally significant is that the 'nursing process' represents only an instrument for practice and perhaps, as yet, can no more represent a theoretical framework for nursing than a 'teaching process' could for education. Nevertheless the emergent 'nursing process' will need careful consideration in any plan for a curriculum, as there is an increasing commitment to its use both in America and the United Kingdom. As a practice-based profession, nursing will for the immediate future continue to draw on those sciences which have been recognised by many nurses as basic to understanding what nurses do for patients and the necessary 'interactions' and interrelationships involved. This is not to say that those things which constitute the delivery and content of nursing (the carrying out of nursing) and the necessary account of individual circumstances in which they take place are not important, for they are. Yet any acceptance of the claim that nursing is a practice-based profession must lead to the assumption that theories in nursing must be interlocking (not merely related) to that practice. This has very important implications for the nursing curriculum, for if theory is to be seen to grow out of practice as well as being a source of direction to practice, professional nurses must have, and go to, the theoretical base of their discipline to obtain a fundamental foundation for realistic curriculum development.

(v) Towards a Conceptual Framework for Nursing

The concern for theory development in nursing is now directing nurses to place emphasis on the development of conceptual frameworks to shape up the emerging theories to some form of logical system. Duffey and Mullenkamp (1974) have stressed that it is through theory development that a scientific body of knowledge emerges and crystallises. Theory has also been seen to provide frameworks which interlock concepts relevant to a particular discipline and both set and order knowledge within the discipline concerned. If then the theoretical base of a discipline also provides the professional foundation for practice and research, as Dickoff and James (1968), Reilly (1975) and McFarlane (1977) indicate, then nursing as a practical discipline must concern itself with theoretical frameworks that will help the nurse use relevant knowledge to guide her actions in the sense that Ellis (1973), Hardy (1974) and McKay (1973) have related the quality of nursing to the level of the individual practitioner's knowledge and understanding.

Whilst it can be seen that there is a concern to develop a body of nursing knowledge, many of the emergent theories lack data of sufficient refinement that allow validation of their assumptions as structures that are likely to guide and shape nursing in reality. In consequence many nurses have difficulty in making practical applications of these theories to practical patient care in clinical settings. Yet nursing as a practical discipline should continue to direct itself to the development of theory that will allow the nurse not only to use knowledge to guide nursing actions, but also to be able to contribute to an incremental development of new knowledge on which to base future practice. It is this form of thinking which has led nurses to consider conceptual and theoretical frameworks in which to base both nursing practice and inquiry. As the most substantial headway has been made in the United States of America, the most notable of these will now be reviewed here.

The growth of nursing theory in the USA is founded in the early historical links of nursing education at a professional level to the university system, which in Great Britain has been a much later and fairly recent development. Although modern nursing began in England with the foundation of the Nightingale School at St Thomas's Hospital, London, in 1860, a look at the English scene today is a look at the

American system of yesterday. McCloskey (1981) sees the nursing conditions in England as similar to those in the United States a generation ago, characterised by low salaries, rigid working conditions, education placed in the hospitals and the nursing service implicitely controlled by physicians.

Certainly today, the emphasis is very much directed to an occupational service ideal which tends to place nursing education in a secondary position of importance. Nurses in Great Britain have as a whole been inadequately remunerated and inadequately recognised as a major caring profession. Without doubt the emphasis on service to the employing authority in respect of student nurses has been the most singularly important deterrent to securing an adequate educational system in nursing. The emphasis on service is also one of the root causes of the profession's inability on previous occasions to establish a foundation of science for nursing. Until there is a concentrated development of methodology that can adequately measure standards of care within the parameters of the basic craft and technology of nursing, standards of care on both sides of the Atlantic will remain subjective and speculative and as such a comparative analysis is only superficially productive. However, contemporary nursing in America does reflect its society's high regard for 'science'. The values of science are easily discernible in the nursing courses and affect the character of its research, education and practice. Nursing dialogue is influenced by technical language, operational definitions, scientific linguistic use of constructs, theories, methodology of scientific enquiry and emphasis on measurement and quantification. Similarly, curriculum standardisation movements as early as 1896 and the Curriculum Committee of the National League of Nursing in 1917 helped steer an early course for curriculum rationalisation in America, producing links with university-based nursing programmes and a spring-board for advancement in nursing theory. Anderson's (1981) analytic review of the historical development of American nursing education reveals that as early as 1927 the NLN had published *A Standard Curriculum for Schools of Nursing*. This book contained concrete suggestions on how to improve standards in the schools of nursing and provided guidelines on how to set up actual courses. It was revised as *A Curriculum for Schools of Nursing*, which also included advances in nursing theory in the intervening decade and emphasised public health, prevention of diseases and sociology. These had been incorporated into good nursing courses as early as the mid-1920s. A third edition called *A Curriculum Guide for Schools of Nursing* was published in 1937. Anderson (1981, p. 31) also shows that at the end of World War II all the national nursing organisations set up planning committees which outlined objectives and defined areas in nursing that needed study. The idea of rational planning and the use of 'curriculum theory' in nursing gained considerable ground in the USA in the two decades following World War II, and nurses were quick to make use of the emerging general curriculum movement fostered by Ralph Tyler and his contemporaries.

It was in the early 1960s, however, that nursing theory began to gather its real momentum in the USA and progressively throughout the 1960s and the 1970s nursing theories and curriculum theory became increasingly established on the nursing educational scene. In a recent analysis, Wu (1979) restated the major problems when she asked: 'What is nursing? What facts, concepts, statements of relationships are relevant to practice in nursing? How is man, society and health conceptualised by nursing?' (p. 16). There had been many attempts to define nursing and it had been variously conceptualised as an 'inter-personal process' (Orlando, 1961), as 'supporting the development process' (Erickson, 1959), 'assisting the individual in the performance of those activities contributing to health or its recovery that would be performed unaided if the necessary strength or knowledge were at hand' (Henderson, 1966), as 'a problem solving process' (Abdellah, 1965), as 'supporting the adaptive process' (Roy, 1976), as 'maintaining behavioural stability' (Johnson, 1968a), and as 'health care' (Schoelfeldt, 1972).

The most significant theorists of this period were Henderson (1966), who distinguished fourteen components of basic nursing care, concentrating on the 'nature of nursing', Abdellah (1965) with 'twenty one nursing problems', Johnson (1968b) with 'eight behavioural systems', Rogers (1970) with a 'model of unitary man', King (1970) with a 'systems approach to nursing', Roy (1976) with an 'adaption model', Orem (1971) with 'man and self-action care' within a systems approach, and Orlando (1961) and Wiedenbach (1964) with emphasis on 'interaction'. King, Orem, Rogers and Roy all see man as the unifying focus of their theories and this unifying focus is seen as central to nursing practice, research and the development of nursing curricula. With each of these theorists although there is basic agreement and similarities in their intent, there are differences in approach, development and content. These similarities and differences have been carefully analysed by McFarlane (1980) who sees the similarities as those of substance and the differences as those of emphasis and semantics (p. 18). My own observations and no doubt those of others lead me to think that these theories, broadly speaking, fall into two generic groups. One can be represented by a systems model and the other group by an interactionist model. The former are represented by Roy's, Rogers' and Johnson's thinking which tends to emphasise 'system' as universal taking account of interdependencies and inherent interactions. The latter are represented by King's, Orem's, Orlando's and Wiedenbach's thinking which appears to emphasise 'gestalt' principles of the whole being greater than the sum of its parts. Here wholeness is the major construct and the individualised care of the patient is the goal of nursing. The major characteristics of the interactionist model have been identified by Bush (1979) as social systems, interpersonal relationships, interactive processes, perceptions and health. Bush (*op. cit.*, p. 20) also identifies a third major group of theoretical models which she calls the 'developmental model' which represents ideas taken from the theoretical works of Freud (1922), Erickson (1959), Maslow (1970) and Rogers (1951). The central theme here is the relationship to growth, development and change to meet stated objectives which take account of the natural and environmental forces within which nursing practitioners work to predict and control the delivery of nursing care. Whatever these theories are, however, in terms of substances, if the central intention is to provide real guidance for nursing practice, it must be tested and validated and the conceptualisations require much more general agreement and a linguistic form which will be meaningful to the day-to-day encounters of the practising nurse.

In contrast to the systems model and the interactionist models, Paterson and Zderad (1976) put forward the idea of 'humanistic nursing'. This is conceptualised as a theory and practice that rests on existentialist philosophy and values experiencing and the evolving of the 'new'. It aims at a phenomenological description of the 'art-science' of nursing viewed as a lived intersubjective transactional experience. In other words, it is nursing seen within its human context. The authors see nursing as both a science and an art form of human responses to human situations and they are valued in genuine humanism. They are careful not to refute nursing technology and the search for scientific theory in nursing, but would try rather to increase the value of such things by viewing their use within the perspective of the development of human potential. Their existentialist view is that every human event and hence every nursing event is unique, a living intersubjective transaction coloured and formed by the individual participants, and that although the event is ephemeral, the resulting experience is knowledge which is lasting and culminative.

Maintaining a humanistic approach to nursing, particularly within health systems that are bureaucratic, is important and the humanistic approach needs to be accounted for. But it is a set of ideals and beliefs rather than an elaborate theory founded on a particular philosophical position that is required in nursing. Duffey and Mullenkamp (1974) remind us that a theory is considered to be hypothetical until enough data are available to support the theory consistently and produce an agreed and 'accepted' addition to the body of knowledge. This means testing hypotheses through research. Dickoff and James (1968) point out the problem as it relates to theory in nursing, when they say that 'theory is born in practice, is refined in research and returns to practice, if research is to be other than a draining off of energy from the main business of nursing, and theory more than idle speculation' (p. 415). The proposals of King (1971), Orem (1971), Roy (1970, 1971) and Rogers (1970) can be seen as conceptual frameworks developed for some purpose, the intention being to guide nursing action and control its outcomes. Yet because the theories need more researched application to actual practice they remain hypothetical at the present time. Is it, therefore, sufficient to look to theory just for definitions, explanations, predictions and so forth? Professional nursing as a practice-based discipline must view the present theories as a series of instruments for structuring, guiding, shaping and controlling patient care in contexts which are pre-eminently nursing and be considered at their most refined as frames for on-going research.

The emphasis so far has been on the North American scene, purely because this is where most theoretical perspectives have been evolved. In the United Kingdom and other West European countries there are relatively few concepts which have been identified with any real sense of assurance. Armstrong-Esther (1979) highlighted the curricula problem for nurses in Britain when he said 'it is clear that our curricula are built from the conventional wisdom of generations of nurses, which is for the most part untested, and conventional wisdom can be a euphemism for ritual, superstition, speculation and unstructured experience.' Certainly the ritualistic procedure orientation of hospital nursing which preceded the 'nursing process' in the USA and is still normative practice in the UK, bears witness to this statement. Similarly, Crow (1981) has viewed the present state of nursing theory (and I suspect on both sides of the Atlantic) as sheer speculation and conjecture based on broad generalisations. She refers to these collectively as constructs, and as these constructs do not appear to have been put to the rigours of scientific testing, they can only be said to represent ideas at the general level of speculation. Although clearly she is not de-bunking nursing theory and would see conjecture as possibly a useful way of characterising the nature of nursing, she makes a strong warning about the dangers of accepting dogmatic arguments which can emanate from hard-line acceptance of speculative models of nursing. Hence, one is led to think that emerging theories cannot be authoritative or even followed as normative practice; they must remain open to criticism, discussion and debate. For as Crow argues, there are rules to obey if nurses want their constructs to be judged as scientific. It is also judgements made by professionals outside nursing that will in the end probably determine whether nursing is recognised as a profession or not. The significant emerging perspective is that nursing theories must eventually be subjected to valid test procedures through deliberate attempts to falsify them in order to secure knowledge that is as objective as possible within the bounds of clinical reality.

It can be seen from the above observations that the present state of nursing theory is in its early, often faltering steps of development. A slow growth of validated hypotheses will no doubt continue to develop over time as the research focus sharpens towards the more significant problems and issues in nursing. But what of the nursing curriculum meantime? How can it take useful account of the present undifferentiated state of nursing knowledge in order to affect the preparation of students of nursing today? A new statutory body for nursing in the UK (The Central Council for Nurses, Midwives and Health Visitors, 1981) is at the time of writing establishing itself in its organisational context. One of its cardinal operational activities will be direction, control and maintenance of a re-shaped educational system for nurses, characterised from recommendations both implicit and explicit within the 'Briggs Report' (1972). Consequently, an innovative paradigm for nursing education in Great Britain may well develop to form the foundation of a new national system for the preparation of nurses in the 1980s.

This new system must have a curriculum or be based on a curricular model that allows flexibility to accommodate a 'developing' body of knowledge and changing professional attitudes, commitments and practices, reflecting what will be a continuous change period for nursing over the two decades into the 21st century. Three assumptions regarding the theoretical arguments for nursing will be attitudinally significant for nurse educators influencing the curricular design. First is an emphasis on concepts and theory as tools for nurses, very much related to nurses seeing the need for nursing practice to be self-initiated, self-contained and self-directed. Secondly, theory in a practical discipline must have application in the sense that 'practice-theory' is considered as thinking intended for nusing action and that professional nursing practice be regarded as activity guided by scientific thinking. Thirdly, nursing research must be used to alter nursing practice and educational activity and nurses must be trained and educated to operate within such changing professional practices. During what will be a continuous period of change for nursing over the next two decades, an adequate and continuous supply of nurses will be required to provide the direct nursing care needed during illness, whether patients are in hospital, the community or some other specialised facility. To meet these commitments nurses must be proficient and accountable for their nursing actions at an increasing level of sophistication in the artistic, scientific and technological senses of nursing practice. A thorough basic knowledge and ability to apply knowledge of those sciences that are seen to underpin nursing practice, i.e. the physical, biological, social and behavioural sciences, is required. The new emerging theoretical perspectives that are distinctively nursing in the 'unique' sense (i.e. the 'nursing process') would be accommodated into the curriculum as an incrementally developing 'core' framework for the curriculum, and be used to make direct applications to the 'on-going' nursing currently operational in the clinical settings. Within the operational curriculum, nurse educators will need to communicate more effectively the distinctive purpose of nursing and to secure the necessary unity of theory and practice, and have an awareness that the ultimate purpose of nursing theory is to inform effective professional nursing practice. As such, the structure and content of the curriculum should seek to communicate an understanding of nursing theory to the student. The quality of the future nursing service may well depend upon the way the educators make effective use of nursing theory, the way it is seen or not seen in relationship to practice, and how nursing knowledge is transmitted through the curriculum.

2 NURSING MODELS AND THEIR RELATIONSHIP TO THE NURSING CURRICULUM

(i) Introduction

Conceptually the word 'model' refers to a precise replication of an object such as a building or a ship. It is also used to abstract an ideal such as a 'model nurse' or a 'model student' or a 'model society', in which case ideals are abstractly conceptualised in advance to demonstrate the feasibility and possibility that such an ideal might be a reality.

Brodbeck (1969) has referred to an intent to be structurally true to the object for which something is a model. Thus the importance of structural truth is that the reality replicated determines the nature of the model and as such the reality is maintained in the model by its form and relationship between its various components. Such model representations can be seen to provide a means of exhibiting, examining and observing the components as structures and relationships of a particular reality. The model can also be adopted as a means of observing, ordering, clarifying and analysing structures, relationships and events, and the process of model construction allows existing knowledge and events to be ordered or re-ordered, conceptualised and understood.

The terms 'model' and 'theory' have been used quite wrongly by some nurses as interchangeable terms. This has led to confusion and restricted to some extent the degree of objectivity the model maker or theorist seeks to attain. The relationship between models and theories is very subtle, but there are clear and necessary distinctions which need to be drawn in order to pursue a logical and objective usage. A model primarily expresses and focuses on structure and inter-relationships rather than on the detailed substance of its subject matter. In doing so it attempts to simplify events by ordering, clarifying and analysing the logical relationships, conceptualisations and general thought elements. The intended outcome is to give unity to the central elements of knowledge in the most economic way with the provision of a main structure and a minimum of detailed content. It is in this way that Batey (1977) sees models as providing a structure or 'map' which enables theory to take form in relation to on-going research (p. 19).

Models are important instruments for nursing theory and practice and assist in the identification of knowledge which can be used by nurses in making curricular arrangements for the transmission of that knowledge in the preparation of new nursing practitioners. It is important that the emerging knowledge which forms the field of study for nurses is set in order, systemised once it is validated and accepted for use in professional practice. This ultimately means that the educational arrangements mediated through the curriculum must be seen as systematic and rational, demonstrating logic and order. There is a need in nursing education to make use of nursing models and curriculum models to develop the best possible arrangements for the education and training of nurses.

(ii) Curriculum Models in Nursing Education

Curriculum models for nursing education can be used in a number of ways. Models have to a greater extent concentrated on guiding teacher and student interactions, planning curricula, selecting suitable materials and evaluating curricula. Models have also been used to unify, direct and simplify educational arrangements and the nurse educator has used them to identify priorities and help focus on the central core of nursing knowledge within an appropriate frame of reference. Models have also been used to identify the baseline of knowledge for the study of nursing, which is variously a selection of topics taken from the biological and behavioural sciences.

In the United States two major groups of models have dominated nurse education and reflect the curricular arrangements for many nursing courses. They are (1) 'general models' that take account of the teaching-learning process and (2) 'specific nursing models' which have been developed to give a theoretical view of nursing as an activity. Examples of nursing specific models used in nursing curricula are Rogers' (1970) model of unitary man, Newman and Young's (1972) total-person approach to patient problems, Roy's (1976) adaptation model and Johnson's (1968b) behavioural systems model.

Rogers' dominant theme is an attempt to conceptualise nursing's aims and goals and focuses on the idea of professional practice. Newman's approach is holistic, while Roy's formalises four models of adaptation as central purposes of nursing. Roy sees the main objectives of nursing as promoting man's adaptation in illness and health with the intent that nursing is identified as a set of adaptive responses. Johnson's approach is through the use of systems theory and she conceptualises nursing as maintaining equilibrium or re-establishing equilibrium within a health-illness dimension. Reduction of stress and tension and promoting adaptation and stability are central intentional elements in Johnson's model.

Shaw (1902), a contemporary of Florence Nightingale, like Nightingale related nursing to health and disease. Shaw also stressed the art of nursing (*op. cit*, pp. 13-14) and viewed nursing as set within interpersonal themes and included a conceptualisation of the nurse-patient relationship. Harmer (1922), like Shaw, emphasised Nightingale's notions of nursing and saw nursing rooted in the needs of humanity and founded on the ideal of service. Within the Harmer model the idea of developing patient independency is clearly seen. Orem (1971) concentrates on the development of 'self-care' which is self-directed or involves the patient learning self-direction in daily self-care. Orem (p. 41) views nursing as a 'family, personal and community service'. She relates the 'nursing process' to the objectives of nursing and nursing goals (p. 157). Abdellah *et al.* (1960) focus on the idea of the nurse as an agent helping people sick or well to cope with their health needs. For Abdellah and her co-workers, nursing is a service to individuals, to families and therefore to society (*ibid.* p. 24). Their model is built on five elements: (1) human relations skills; (2) observation and communication in reporting signs and symptoms and deviations from normal behaviour; (3) interpretation of observations to identify deviations from health as nursing problems; (4) analysis of the nursing problem and selection of appropriate actions; and (5) organisation of the nurses' effort to achieve nursing results by helping the patient to return to health (p. 26). Abdellah includes a typology of nursing problems to be solved which focus on the physical, biological and social needs of the patient. The Abdellah model is very much in tune with the idea of nursing being a process, with the nurse clearly involved in information processing and problem solving. The broad knowledge base in most of these models can be seen to be eclectic and there is an obvious readiness to draw from several disciplines in the search for concepts and techniques which will make sense for individual patients, rather than insisting that all patients and their problems are interpreted within the confines of one theoretical system.

In the United Kingdom, Roper (1976) has proposed a model of nursing based on a model of living to assist in the development of a conceptual structure for nursing. From her Scottish based study, the intention was to use the model as a base, from which a discipline of nursing could develop. Influenced by Hirst (1968), Roper sees the discipline of nursing as a 'nursology' with characteristic modes of thinking that would allow the following of a dictum. In this context nurses would be trained and educated to 'think nursologically' (Roper 1976, p. 83). A distinctive body of knowledge characterised by nursology models of thinking would eventually allow nurses to put nursing among the learned disciplines. Roper's model is based on 'activities of daily living', within which the central assumptions are that the model of living has a life span on a dimension from conception to death and the living person is modelled as requiring help with or partaking of four groups of activities. These groups of activities are, namely, (1) daily living, (2) preventing, (3) comforting, and (4) seeking activities. Nursing is therefore represented as comprising four groups of components based on the model of living's four groups of activities. Objectives are used and the activities of daily living components are performed and stand in individual relationship to each patient or client in a health care system. As such they are concerned with either acquisition, maintenance or restoration of maximum independence, or assistance, so that patients can cope with being dependent in any of the activities of daily living.

Most of the nursing specific models can be seen to focus as clinical models and have to a greater or lesser extent been based on assumptions taken from some existing prototype theories such as 'developmental adaptation' and 'interaction theories' and re-represented as particular views of what nursing is about.

(iii) Curriculum Models in Nursing

Most curriculum models in nursing tend to follow a fairly distinctive form. Chater (1975) views this distinctiveness in a 'three component approach' represented by specific attention to the student, the school or faculty, and the subject matter. Thus, emphasis is placed on context, content and the individual. The student component tends to take account of knowledge of student characteristics including motivational theories, educational level, goals, interests, self and social roles. These are subsumed through appropriate teaching-learning approaches. The second component concentrates on issues and problems related to the school and hospital environment and takes account of the organisational and contextual interrelationships. The third component is concerned with selection of content with the emphasis placed on knowledge, skills and attitudes. It is usually this third component that attempts to make use of theoretical definitions of nursing and particular views and beliefs about the activity of nursing practice by using a model such as the 'nursing process'. It is also this component that is most problematic for it often incorporates a specific nursing model (or models) by which description and prescription of the nature of nursing is perceived for curricula purposes.

For instance, Derdiarian (1979) focuses on discussing goals for nursing practice and education by relating some common nursing intentions to models of nursing. She argues for a subscription to the goals of nursing practice and for a 'core' content of nursing as dictated by nursing models (p. 39). This approach can be difficult for the curriculum designer concentrating on 'core' content for nursing programmes because of the multiplicity of available models and a general lack of conceptual agreement and common frames of reference.

Peterson (1977), with this problem in mind, proposed a series of questions and propositions which usefully identify elements of nursing content:

(1) What is the nature of the service being provided to the client (patient) – that is, how do you describe nursing?
(2) What is the goal or outcome to which the service is directed – that is, how do you view health and well-being?
(3) Why does the client need the services nursing provides?
(4) How do you describe the giver of the service – the nurse? Is she/he a professional or technical practitioner?
(5) How is the client described?
(6) How do you describe the context for the services?

This form of self-questioning may help direct thinking to the identification of the important elements of a conceptual framework which would then take into account the patient, the nurse, social health care interactions and the nature of nursing care delivery within a total social environment.

Meleis (1979) sees both forms of modelling (nursing-specific and curricular) as the most useful approach to the development of a conceptual framework, and as such they can be viewed as complementary in the development of nursing curricula (p. 664). It would appear that there is a relatively well developed consensus of opinion about the need for a nursing model or multi-models to help represent the process (how nursing is carried out) and the content (what nursing is) as a framework for professional practice. There is undoubtedly an equal need for a curriculum model to help ensure that the process and content of nursing receive effective educational delivery to students of nursing.

Perhaps the nursing-specific models can be seen to shape and direct the process and content of nursing which reflects nursing practice. The curriculum models would similarly give guidance and operational direction for the nursing educational and training agreements, by providing sharper and more critical attention to selection and ordering of knowledge and learning experiences for the student of nursing. It might be useful at this stage to examine the relationship of conceptual frameworks to curriculum models and to seek a distinction between each of these on the assumption that a useful distinction can be made.

(iv) Conceptual Frameworks and Curriculum Models

In relationship to the curriculum for nursing, Torres and Yura (1974) have defined a conceptual framework as a representation of the faculty's (schools) notions or symbols that give structure to the curriculum so that its parts can be fitted and united into the total programme. Such a framework provides a rationale for the selection of learning experiences and a system for classifying knowledge of the conceptual or theoretical field. Wu (1979) looks at the model as a symbolic representation of the real world of nursing and, accepting that there are different kinds of models, sees nursing curricula most closely resembling a descriptive model rather than an iconic (pictorial) model in the sense that it focuses primarily on the structure of conceptual relationships (p. 14).

Certainly, a model representing the nursing curriculum is structurally similar to a conceptual framework as defined by Torres and Yura, for it is a representation of the real world, that is, in this instance the world of nursing. The curriculum model is seen to be providing a rationale for the selection of learning experiences and provision of structures for identifying and ordering information and is more likely to allow the correct set and sequences of knowledge to provide essential unity. The difference, as Wu (*ibid.*) points out, is in the purposes defined for each. For instance, the purpose of the curriculum model is to ensure that things such as aims and goals are congruent with the known requirements of the student and the nursing requirements of the patients in the health care system of a society. Subsequently, the components are so interrelated that the end result or outcome is a professional nurse that functions in accordance with the intent of the model. It achieves this by providing a structure for the organisation of learning experiences which includes the identification of the antecedent and specific knowledge of nursing and their correct or most useful sequences and relationships. The activities therein are guided by the model and as such a curriculum in action, or the curriculum process at work, can be designed from it.

In contrast to the curriculum model, the conceptual framework of the curriculum is concerned with how various ideas and symbolic representations relate to each other to produce a holistic effect. Torres and Yura (1974) see most nursing curricula organised by relevance to a conceptual framework. Their conceptual framework encompasses at least four elements: (1) the individual; (2) society; (3) health; and (4) nursing. Using elements such as these a conceptual framework sets certain parameters and guidelines which can be used as points of reference for nursing practice. Such frames of reference provide a theoretical perspective and an organisational structure for dealing with the curricular implications of such important aspects of nursing as the 'nursing process' and its effects upon patient care and patient behaviour. Within the boundaries of such a framework certain major concepts can be identified and developed, such as: (1) role; (2) self-concept; (3) health and illness; (4) communication; (5) nursing care delivery. Theories can then be selected for the curriculum that will give the clearest explanations and most meaningful interpretation of these concepts.

Whatever framework is ultimately adopted, the individual patient and the individual nurse would be seen in terms of their needs, motivation, growth and development patterns, and focus on how these elements influence the various actions and responses in the interaction of nursing care. In addition to this interactive element of nursing which is the essence of 'care', the conceptual framework would need to take account of the family group, the work group and their related social norms, other professional groups in health care, political, economic and other social regulating influences. All of these have influences on what nurses do, and how they do it, in the context of nursing care provision – and they require study and analysis as likely selections for the curriculum. Within this form of framework, hypotheses can be generated concerning the interactions between the individual and the social system, involving health as a particular 'state of being', and a dimension of health from minimal to optimal states can be analysed.

(v) The 'Nursing Process' as a Co-ordinating Element in the Nursing Curriculum

Systematic approaches to detecting and analysing patients' nursing and health needs and establishing goals that are harmonious with their patterns of daily living and adapting and planning care accordingly are a new central element in nursing practice. This central element is usually identified as the process of nursing or the 'nursing process', and it embraces the specific skills of scientific method or problem-solving. This particular attempt at systematising nursing care is increasingly believed to be basic to all clinical nursing practice and is now receiving world-wide recognition.

Simms (1973) sees the process as operational skills in clinical nursing practice and lists the following which are considered as primary skills (p. 95).

(1) To make an assessment of the nursing problem, using all available, relevant data about the patient.
(2) To establish goals or objectives for the nursing regimen.
(3) To design the plan of nursing care.
(4) To develop and prescribe nursing actions to implement the plan of care.
(5) To observe, analyse and evaluate the results of nursing actions in terms of the goals and plan of care.
(6) To make adaptations in any of the steps as indicated.
(7) To record and report the process and results in a systematic way.

Simms (p. 96) argues for mastery of interviewing skills, discriminative skills, teaching skills, collaborative skills, leadership skills and skills in writing. The nursing process and communication skills constitute the intellectual element of nursing care in Simms' analysis. Interviewing skills are required to learn about the patient and his problem, discriminative skills to observe the patient, teaching skills for self-care, collaborative skills to collaborate with other health professionals in planning care, leadership skills for teamwork and linguistic skills for continuity of care.

The 'nursing process' has been described in a number of ways but, within most definitions, a logical sequence is always revealed within which the nurse seeks to provide systematic care based on rational thinking and action. King (1970) analyses the process as a series of acts which she calls action, reaction and interaction. These are said to be followed by a transaction when a reciprocal relationship has been established. In such a transaction both nurse and patient are active participants in determining goals to be achieved in the nursing care. King sees the transaction from the nurse's point of view as assisting the individual patient irrespective of age or socio-economic group to meet his basic needs in performing activities of daily living and to cope with health and illness at particular points in the life cycle (p. 91). Mayers (1978) stresses skills in the nursing process as being technical, behavioural and intellectual and based on theories and principles derived from physical and social sciences (p. 4). Also in Mayers' account, sequence and logic are made apparent in her description of the phases of the process. The phases are seen to be interrelated and recycling in nature and are represented as data-gathering (assessment), problem identification (diagnosing), goal determination (predicted patient outcomes), intervention planning (prescribing), plan implementation (direct or indirect care), and evaluation which is concurrent and retrospective (p. 244).

It is clear that the process is viewed as dynamic and problem solving and four main stages are constant in most accounts. The four stages are *assessment*, *planning*, *implementation and evaluation*, and the process seeks to individualise nursing care. The assessment stage is concerned with identifying the problems and the needs of the patient and is followed by analysis and information processing whereby relevant data are brought to light that have bearing on the patient's care. The planning stage follows the assessment and may be preceded by deciding specific nursing objectives. A care plan is drawn up in accordance with the objectives. The implementation stage is the actual intervention or delivery of nursing care. In the last stage, evaluation is carried out by which the value of care is determined. The process is usually seen as a continuous cycle of events rather than as a simple linear approach.

Altschul (1978) uses a systems approach to the nursing process, based on problem-solving and activities of daily living. Norton (1981) has called the nursing process 'the quiet revolution' in nursing and likens it to a philosophy which is uniquely nursing (p. 1069). She also stresses the importance of objectives preceding the planning stage (p. 1069). McCarthy (1981) has explored the relationship of the nursing process to clinical problem-solving in the literature of medicine and sees the process as having 'fit' with current research thoughts on decision-making in nurses' work. Smeltzer (1980), similarly, sees practical method within the nursing process, also stresses objectives and argues that the process could form a conceptual framework for the curriculum. Sculco (1978) also has the process as an integral part of the curriculum for purposes of organisation and development of clinical objectives (p. 41), and she argues perceptively for the differentiation of objectives, with the presentation of a taxonomy.

Using the nursing process approach to care in the curriculum can be dealt with at various levels of simplicity and sophistication. At a very basic and simplistic level the process can be introduced and discussed in terms of its application to individual patients. In this context, nursing care planning is studied and the nursing care plan is explained as an instrument for assisting the application of the nursing process. The idea of a standard care plan can be introduced to show how the nursing process can be applied to a particular patient or health problem. Individual personalised adaptations to a standard care plan can be made, the detailed adaptations being dependent on the individual variables related to the patient, his social and health values. The focus of learning for the students is on comprehension and application of the nursing process to relatively simple nursing contexts.

At an intermediate level of curricular application, the nursing process can be treated at a higher level of complexity, in situations where health and patient problems are less obvious, more complex and the technical, behavioural and social skills application more advanced. In this instance, the nursing process is accounted for in a learning environment requiring 'in depth' applications which make greater cognitive, affective and psycho-motor demands on the student nurse. This intermediate level of difficulty reinforces the early learning of the process at the basic level by the students. In essence, they move on a stage to master formulation of their own standard care plans to analyse critically and evaluate their effectiveness. The individual creativity of the student is encouraged at this stage by seeking to develop skills in prediction, analysis and evaluation as further sophistications of the cognitive aspect of problem-solving.

The nursing process can also be used in the curriculum at an advanced level of sophistication. At this level, new and broader dimensions can be added in such a way as to prepare the nurse for increased individual professional responsibility through planning, decision-making and leadership exercises. At this advanced level of study the nursing process is used within a theoretical frame of reference from which the student can formulate nursing care plans that reflect various and sometimes differing theories of health and disease. The analysis of individual patient situations from several theoretical positions is required with an ultimate goal of developing plans of care based on theory that is seen as most relevant to a particular care context. In this way, the student develops abilities in the discriminative and synthetic use of patient data and makes the most relevant application of planned nursing care to both individuals and groups in general or specialised contexts.

By using three levels of application of the nursing process within a particular course or modular unit there is a gradual development of the process from simplistic to advanced, and comprehensive learning experiences can be developed for the student. In this way, student learning is progressive through the increasing development of the skills required. Prediction, discrimination, synthesis and evaluation abilities are developed through skilled analysis. This spiral and cyclic use of the process continuously reinforces the student's ability to use it in varying contexts, and the nursing process develops as a curricular theme and a co-ordinating element within the curriculum as a whole.

Much has been written in praise of the nursing process and the new Central Council for Nursing, Midwifery and Health Visiting is using it in the current draft syllabuses for Mental Nursing and Mental Subnormality Nursing (1981). It is, however, important to see the nursing process from a realistic point of view and to be careful not to expect it to function as some sort of panacea for all the answers to the theory-practice dilemma. A common assumption that the nursing process is *the* theory of nursing is both dangerous and, in the long run, non-productive as far as securing a unique body of knowledge is concerned. It would indeed be a mistake dogmatically to hang emerging theories of nursing onto a process model. It would be no more logical to do this, than it would to represent all research on the 'scientific model' to the exclusion of all others, or to represent all management theory as the 'management process' of all pedagogical theory as a 'teaching process', or all learning theory as a 'learning process'. The nursing process in its present form is a useful instrument which will help nurses rationalise and organise nursing care on patient-centred individual approaches. The theoretical and practical activities of nursing (nursing knowledge) should not be subordinated to one process approach, because the process is no more than an element of the whole. Nevertheless, it is a vital element and one that requires careful application and recognition within the overall scheme of things for nursing education.

(vi) The Use of Curriculum Theory and Practice in Nursing Education

The nursing curriculum reform movement most notable in the United

States of America and increasingly in the United Kingdom is influenced to a great extent by curriculum theorists in general education, particularly Tyler (1950), Taba (1962), Bloom (1956) and Mager (1967). Objective approaches to learning outcomes in many nursing programmes are readily seen in the work of Bolvin (1968), Baker and Goldberg (1970), Pletsch (1979), Reilly (1975), Dyer (1979) and Greaves (1980). Similarly, systems approaches taking considerable account of objectives can be seen in the work of Flint (1980), Griggs (1977), Sullivan (1977), and Harms and McDonald (1966) and systems evaluation by Boe (1980).

Linked to both objective and systems approaches is the idea of the individualisation of learning using instructional perspectives leading to the mastery of material. These approaches have been argued for by Baker and Goldberg (1970), Bolvin (1968), Corona (1979) and Notter and Robey (1979). Individuality is linked to a mastery of learning concepts and learning is viewed as a continuous progress within the curriculum. In this form of approach, Olsen (1979) has critically analysed a competence-based curriculum which was seen as a precision-refinement of the objectives model, emphasising mastery, individuality and accountability in nursing practice.

Integration of content in the curriculum has also received considerable attention from Wu (1979), Hipps (1981), Jaffee *et al*. (1979), Parsons (1980) and Levine (1979). These authors have concentrated on integrative factors, inter-relatedness, scope and sequencing of content as curricular design approaches.

The nursing process as a curricular inclusion is now receiving considerable support as an integral design feature. The nursing process as a systems model has been proposed by Christman and Riehl (1974) and by Brown (1980) and the process is seen as important, if not central, to the curriculum by Miller (1980), Welch and Slagle (1980), Smeltzer (1980) and Whelton (1979).

Philosophical attention to the nursing curriculum is also being considered, but to a much lesser extent. Weitzel (1980) has stressed the necessity of a philosophical input, and Dickoff and James (1970) have considered at length a beliefs and values base for the nursing curriculum. Generally speaking, the philosophical approaches tried have been too holistic and more second order forms of discussion are required from the philosophical standpoint.

The most fruitful area of endeavour in nursing curricula is the now agreed need for conceptual bases and from a design point of view is seen in the work of the National League of Nursing (1974), characterised through the approaches of Torres and Yura (1974), Chater (1975), Moritz (1979) and Orem (1971). A further central area of concern is seen in relationship to change and change-processes as they affect the development of the curriculum and implementation of the curriculum. Williamson (1976) and Novello (1976) have recognised and illuminated the changing nursing scene as critically important for nursing education; and Dyer (1979), Ketefian (1978) and Greaves (1982) have related change-process variables such as attitude, decision-making and implementation factors of innovations as they affect the operationalisation of the curriculum.

It is clear that much attention is currently being given to nursing curriculum design on both sides of the Atlantic and that curriculum theory and skills derived from it are becoming prerequisites for effective course design and evaluation. Within the present growth of the nursing curricular reform movement it is essential to take account of the models of nursing, conceptual frameworks and general curriculum theory, for the following reasons:

(1) The existence of a logically integrated body of knowledge is often assumed by curriculum workers, planners and developers and this assumption may be unrealistic.
(2) Nursing considered as a field of knowledge is generally speaking poorly organised for curricular outcomes.
(3) Curriculum planners are in danger of being overwhelmed by the potential scope and diversity of the knowledge requirements for effective nursing and by the unorganised state of nursing knowledge.
(4) Any in-depth approach to curriculum design, development and evaluation requires consideration and debate of both nursing models and a curriculum model.

3 CURRICULUM THEORY AND PRACTICE: PLANNING APPROACHES – THE CURRICULAR PROCESS

(i) Introduction

Curriculum development in a planned rational sense is new to nursing education in the United Kingdom. This is not a surprising state of affairs, as it is only over the last two decades that it has received serious attention in the field of general education. The nursing curriculum in the past has to a large extent developed in a somewhat haphazard manner without much consideration given to any developmental process. Consequently the curriculum has been devoid of objectivity and outdated both in content and methodology. Adjustments to content and method have been carried out usually in a piecemeal fashion over time as latent responses to new social and health care demands. The outcome of this for nursing education has been a rather static curriculum and an increasing departure from the question of relevance. Much of the curriculum has continued to be dominated by traditional modes of thinking with the craft aspect of nursing emphasised without adequate supporting theory, and inconsistent relationships between new nursing practice, research and education. It has to be recognised that an effective nursing curriculum will thrive only on its degree of relevance to the present realities in nursing and the extent to which the nursing curriculum is capable of assisting the student of nursing to succeed in nursing. This means that the nursing curriculum cannot effectively operate in a vacuum. If students are to be properly prepared for occupational competence and accountability in professional nursing, the curricular focus must be concerned with relevance and mastery of content by the student developed on a basis of what she knows and what she can do.

The curriculum for nursing must set forth the order and scope of what is to be learned to increase the probability that the desired learning will occur. A planned curriculum is required to ensure that the programme offered is consistent with the learning requirements of individual practitioners. In order to have such consistency, use must be made of the theory and practice of the curriculum process itself. Because the curriculum is dynamic in nature rather than static, the dynamic nature has to be accounted for in the planning and organisation which can be best achieved by viewing the curriculum as something that is active and changing. The active curriculum (a curriculum in action) can be effectively developed through the use of an interactive process which allows for clear intentions, unified and relevant content, suitable methods and evaluation.

The nursing curriculum must reject atomisation of its knowledge bases in its subject organisation to reduce the future fragmentation of content. As nursing knowledge is in a rapid growth phase, particularly in its degree of specialisation, a focus of application must be directed ultimately to studying nursing problems in their entirety. This means that the totality of co-ordinated offerings will be dependent on a unified curricular approach. The focus of the content can be its centre of organisation and for the nursing curriculum a major organising focus may well be the nursing process. One of the major weaknesses in the traditional nursing courses is the lack of focus. Whether the curriculum is organised by subjects, topics or by modules, the fluid nature of the curriculum makes it difficult to decide which dimensions are important to pursue, which facts and ideas to emphasise and which to temper down. Using the nursing process as a focal point may within the curricular organisation help preserve and protect both the logic of the content and the psychological sequence of the learning experiences. It seems logical that if unity and focus are important for the content of the curriculum and certain desired learning outcomes are required, organised curricular approaches will help secure greater success in design. The knowledge and skills acquired by the students will be dependent on adequate description and prescription of specific learning experiences to secure adequate internalisation of the content. Certain principles of organisation will be required for successful programming. A successful programme will be one that is carefully and thoughtfully put together in terms of its purpose and clarity of intentions. Goals and objectives will in this respect be important and the expanding body of nursing knowledge will have to be viewed as broad in scope and varied in content and allow a sequence of culminative learning experiences.

(ii) Curriculum Development: A Rational Approach

The word curriculum has only in the last two decades begun to mean more than the content of a syllabus and the programme of course arrangements. To some it has denoted a specific course, while more recently to others it has encompassed the entire educational environment. A general definition could be the sum of learning activities and experiences that a student has under the auspices of the school. Kerr (1968) similarly views the curriculum as 'all the learning planned and guided by the school' (p. 16) and in so doing includes the methods employed, the way in which the school is organised, including the beliefs and values along with social skills which the school intends the student to learn. Kerr (p. 17) also proposes a model of the curriculum which directs attention to the purpose of the curriculum, the subject matter to be used, the learning experiences and organisational contexts and assessment of the results. Four classical curricular elements, therefore, characterise Kerr's approach: objectives, content, methods and evaluation.

Taba (1962), Hooper (1971), Hirst (1975) and Wheeler (1967) support models broadly similar to Kerr's and the attraction of this relatively simple approach is in the suggestion of four basic questions: (i) What is the curriculum's purpose? (ii) What subject matter is to be used? (iii) What learning experiences and school organisation are to be provided? (iv) How are the results to be assessed? Taba (*op. cit.*, p. 14) views curriculum as a rational planned design of educational activities which are calculated to diagnose needs, formulate objectives, select content, organise content, select learning experiences and organise learning experiences. She also sees evaluation and ways and means to evaluate as part of the process. For Taba, curriculum as a developmental activity is rational rather than a rule of thumb procedure and within a rational approach decision-making is required based on orderly thinking so that all relevant considerations are brought to bear on the decisions made. The idea of rationality is central in Taba's thinking when she proposes a theory and practice for curriculum development. Thus she follows a systematic strategy and a step-by-step methodology which allows for logical and ordered planning. She argues for the need not only to follow a rational scheme of planning for the various elements but also to have a method for developing these elements and relating them to each other. The methodological sequence of Taba's approach is very close to a comparable sequence proposed by Tyler (1950). The rationality in Taba's approach, however, is set within a conceptual system for the curriculum which uses theory to organise all the matters that are seen as important to curriculum development. For both Taba and Tyler, their conceptual approach directs the focus of the curriculum designer towards such questions as: what are the important elements of the curriculum? how are they chosen and organised? and how are criteria and information relative to the curriculum elements translated into curricular decisions?

Taba specifies in this sense a statement of curricular design which not only identifies the elements of the curriculum, but also their relationships to each other (*op. cit.*, p. 421). From Taba's specification it is possible to use principles of organisation and specify the administrative conditions under which the curriculum will operate. From Taba's analysis it is clearly seen that planning based on systematic approaches and organisational principles is a prerequisite for effective curriculum design. The question becomes not whether we should plan, but how to plan in the best possible way. This assumption directs curriculum planning to a more scientific approach, that will rationally recognise facts and allow objective considerations, rather than beliefs and personal preferences.

Wheeler (1967), much influenced by Taba's work on curriculum development, has also developed systematic and rational approaches to curriculum problems and has proposed guidelines for curriculum development and evaluation which culminate in a process approach which is proposed as a 'curriculum process'. The process is modelled on five stages which have a cyclic rather than linear relationship (p. 31). Wheeler's five phases are thus considered as sequentially related and interdependent and each phase is considered as a logical development from the preceding one. The five phases are: (i) the selection of aims, goals and objectives; (ii) the selection of learning experiences calculated to help in the attainment of these aims, goals and objectives; (iii) the selection of content (subject matter), through which certain types of experience may be offered; (iv) the organisation and integration of learning experiences and content with respect to the teaching-learning process within school and classroom; (v) evaluation of the effectiveness of all aspects of phases (ii), (iii) and (iv) in attaining the goals detailed in phase (i) (*op. cit.*, p. 30). The distinctive features of Wheeler's model are that curriculum planning is a continuous and on-going activity and includes organisation as a specific stage. Content tends to be selected after learning experiences have been planned and these in turn are chosen to meet specific objectives.

(iii) Intentions and Purposes: An Objective Approach

The importance of objectives in curriculum design has been advocated on and off for many years and there is an extensive literature on the value of their use in curriculum development and evaluation. Among curriculum theorists there is general agreement that intentions and purposes are a necessary stage in the design process. Bobbit (1924), Charters and Waples (1929) and Tyler (1950) were early advocates for the clarification of intentions of the educators' developing programmes. Tyler states that the first question that must be answered in developing a curriculum is: what educational purposes should the school seek to attain? (p. 1). He does tend to use the terms goal, purpose and educational objective interchangeably. For instance, educational programmes should have clearly defined purposes, some conception of the goals that are being aimed at and educational objectives by which materials are selected, content is outlined, instructional procedures developed and tests and examinations prepared (*ibid*., p. 3). Certainly in Tyler's conceptual framework for the curriculum, objectives are meant to stand at the heart of the scheme and very much relate to the intention of bringing about changes in learner behaviour. Davies (1976) develops this theme to its most logical conclusion when he in simple but effective terms says that 'without objectives there is no guarantee that you will know where you are going, nor is there any likelihood that you will recognise when you have arrived (p. 77). For Davies, objectives are important in helping the designer to answer the question: what is the curriculum attempting to achieve? In other words, they force the designer to be clear and precise about the intention within the curriculum. Kemp (1971) takes a more generalised approach and he argues that all educational programmes are based upon broadly stated goals which involve ethical and philosophical considerations. Kemp does differentiate between the terms goal and purpose by stating that goals function as the source for selection of major topics and give direction and emphasis to instructional planning.

Eisner (1979) makes an important contribution in which he stresses the significance of language modification around the word objective (p. 104). Early formulations were educational objectives and this term was shifted by other writers to instructional objectives, later still to behavioural objectives and even later to performance objectives. Eisner argues (p. 105) that this language modification is not accidental, but reflects an increasing emphasis on the behaviour of the student. The shift in emphasis is in fact from the general to the specific to predict and secure educational outcomes. For Eisner this modification of language is not just related to minor differences in linguistic style but is seen as an increasing attempt to secure precision and clarity of intentions.

Mager (1967) can be claimed to have directed the curriculum movement from a position of broad often ambiguous intentions to one of more specific intent. He broke new ground by using specific behavioural objectives and insisting that specific and explicit elements should characterise the use of objectives. Mager clearly saw that when goals are lacking in clarity of intent it becomes impossible to evaluate a course or programme efficiently and there is no sound basis for selecting appropriate materials, content, or instructional method (p. 31). Mager's position on objectives is that the objective is an intent communicated by a statement describing a proposed change in a learner – a statement of what the behaviour is to be like when he has successfully completed a learning experience (*ibid*, p. 131). In other words, it is a description of a pattern of behaviour (performance) we want the learner to be able to demonstrate. There is no doubt that Mager's approach is significantly helpful for teachers in their immediate day-to-day teaching activities. What Mager has shown us is how objectives can reduce the chance of ambiguity and double standards. In this way objectives can be used as the basis for communication between the teacher and learner about what the learner has to learn. They can also be used to prescribe the choice of teaching approach and similarly as a basis for individualised instruction.

The works of Bloom (1956) and Krathwohl, Bloom and Masia (1964) provided the first classification of objectives in the now classical taxonomy. This has set forth a design classification for the intended outcomes of the educational process. The cognitive, affective and later the psychomotor (Harrow, 1972) domains, are now seen to be essentially directing the intended behaviour of students and stressing the relationship of objectives to content, integral organisation and evaluation. The work of Bloom and co-workers and the significant contribution of Mager provide a sound theoretical framework for objective approaches in curriculum design. The critical dimension of a taxonomic system of objectives is its potential for facilitating clearer communication in matters of curriculum planning. It also moves some way to providing an acceptable standard frame of reference to indicate learning outcomes that teachers seek to evaluate. The taxonomy is useful for helping nurse educators develop pre-determined high quality objectives and increases the likelihood of greater intelligent use of objectives. In this sense the taxonomy can aid as a reference frame in the development of a nursing curriculum.

Herrick and Tyler (1950) have argued that curriculum development without the use of curriculum theory is inadequate, and that curriculum theory without development denies the essential purpose of theory. The focus of this argument implies that curriculum theory and practice are inter-dependent and, as such, complementary to each other. The theory and practice of curriculum development has no concept more central to curriculum planning than the concept of objectives. The whole logic of rational planning rests on specifying obtainable objectives and at the present stage of curriculum thinking, behavioural objectives appear to be the only rational approach worked out in sufficient detail to have useful practical application in planning the nursing curriculum.

A major difficulty among nurse educationists concerns the degree of confusion that surrounds such terms as aims, goals and objectives. In order to clarify some of the difficulties, and off-set some of the inconsistencies, the following guide is offered. First, *aims* are broad statements of intent and serve as very broad guidelines, rather than offering a specification. They are frequently seen to be vague, rhetorically formed and over-simplified, though they are valuable for idealising and conceptualising the more cherished educational aspirations in the curriculum, such as quality of nursing care. They often carry a value judgement, indicate broad directions to take in the curriculum by general prescription and recommendation of something. Aims are frequently concerned with general policy, priorities and particular strategy rather than with tacitness or exactness.

Goals are usually found somewhere between aims and objectives; they are more explicit than aims but not as precise as objectives. They often indicate sub-classifications of an aim and focus towards learner outcomes without specifying details of anticipated student performances. The *objective* specifies behaviour that can be seen in student performance, and the objectives are seen as learning outcomes rather than teacher or teaching objectives. In other words the objectives describe what the student will do, not what the teacher will do. The strength of the behavioural objective lies in its potential tactical nature in that it can be made explicitly operational. From a practical point of view a valid objective will describe and prescribe in the clearest possible terms the student activity within the intended learning experience. Writing objectives also disciplines teachers to be clear about their intentions and improves the communication of learning intent to the students.

Teachers may be more accountable if their intentions are clearly known to both themselves and the students and the teacher-learner interactions become more productive. Certainly when objectives are known to students they act as detailed guidelines by informing them, stimulating them and motivating them. In this way, the objectives serve as a form of advanced organiser for independent study.

Nursing curricula in the United Kingdom are already making use of objective approaches. Their use provides for rational planning in the sense that the curriculum planner knows exactly what kind of behaviour he or she wants learners to display. Also it is easier to identify and select content and formulate activities that are instrumental in achieving the desired end – see Quinn (1980), Sheahan (1980) and Greaves (1980).

There are critics of the objectives movement in the curriculum literature. The most notable of these are MacDonald-Ross (1973), Stenhouse (1970), Atkins (1968) and Kneller (1972). Although there is no outright rejection of behavioural objectives, there are several warnings raised about the relationship of objectives to the complex relationships in educational values and prescribed learning outcomes. There is also a risk of total commitment to the utility and instrumental function of the curriculum whereby the content of education can be distorted and misrepresented by dogmatic objective approaches. The current developing objectives approach in the nursing curriculum must be more than simply a paper exercise. There must be an intelligent and sensitive use made of objectives in the nursing curriculum by which creative approaches to the education and training can be nourished and the level of educational excellence increased and maintained. The use of objectives must be directed to this creativity and away from rigid, inflexible and dogmatic approaches.

(iv) Curriculum Content: Organisation and Planning

Three major tasks confront curriculum designers when setting out to build a curriculum. First, the content of the curriculum (the knowledge and skills) have to be described. Secondly, the learning experiences needed by the students to enable the learning of the content to take place have to be identified and planned. Thirdly, the appropriate range and variety of teaching strategies that are deemed appropriate have to be developed. When these tasks have been achieved, a framework of course areas, units and themes have to be created.

There are certain basic principles of curricular organisation that can help in the production of a rational programme in addition to those governed by the aims, goals and objectives. A progressive approach to organisation and planning should be seen as a step by step method which defines and proceeds from means to ends. It begins by defining the ends desired. The means are then selected to obtain best those identified and selected ends and by a series of approximations involving the definition and utilisation of feedback, the process is correctable and is improved with each successive application.

Taba (1962) and Bloom (1958) have characterised their approaches to curriculum through this basically scientific procedure with assumptions based on a means-end orientated view of educational planning. Later important psychological inputs also emerged in the work of Gagné (1965), Glaser (1963), Popham (1969) and Mager (1962), in which the essential elements of planning procedure rested firmly on step-by-step moves that led to ends that are known in advance and the attainment of the desired ends which were to be realised through maximum instructional efficiency. In this classical form of approach, Eisner (1979) sees the central problem of this technological orientation to curriculum not as questioning ends but rather in the planning sense to operationalise them through statements that are referenced to observable behaviour (p. 67). The means-end model of curriculum planning has the virtue of systematising educational planning. It ensures that planners formulate their purposes and allows them to use those purposes as criteria for evaluating the efficiency and effectiveness of the plans that are made. The strategic planning within the model also involves questions of scope, sequence, integration and continuity.

(v) The Importance of Structure: Scope, Sequence, Continuity and Integration

Viewing curriculum design as a set of activities to improve upon the unplanned chance that desired outcomes will be acquired involves considerations of scope and sequence. In this context the design function includes setting forth the order and scope of what is to be taught so that the essential learning may be enhanced. This is essentially a decision-making exercise concerning such things as the outside limits of the content, the way in which it is put together (mapped-out), integrated and given continuity. It involves a particular set of values about the nature of the content and a particular relationship of ideas in its various themes and broad areas. It is also concerned with the balance of the curricular content, its emphasis and central key ideas. It concerns problems of the exclusiveness of certain elements of content, the degree of fusion of subjects, the use of themes or strands and the identification of various paths and trails that should be followed. It involves decisions about the extent of complexity and difficulty and thus is concerned with the modes of learning and the conditions under which learning takes place. In giving consideration to these the designer makes assumptions about the learning stimulated by the curricular arrangements which are influenced by the most effective sequences of curricular events. In other words he takes account of certain concepts and assumptions about how learning takes place and which instructional events are critical for the learning to occur. The designer has in terms of organising the curricular structure to make assumptions concerning certain variables that must be operative to produce the learning outcomes or behaviour changes that the curriculum plan intended. The sequence of instructional events in this respect may be, for a particular designer, a significant aspect of the design, in which case the curriculum will be planned by securing the validity of principles about the interdependence of the learning events. These interdependencies may well be formalised as course sequences emphasising a prescribed order in which the student is exposed to the content and particular instructional events.

Scope

Given that the curriculum includes a design which is itself a series of decisions, the question of what to include poses questions about the scope. These questions are inevitably related to that of 'what criteria?', through which it is necessary to develop a set of criteria that will help in the selection of the content and experiences. These criteria are central in considering what is to be included in the curriculum and this is sometimes collectively referred to as 'determining the scope', or the range of subject matter, content and methodology to be used.

Phenix (1964) relates scope to modes of understanding and offers a schema drawn from disciplined communities of inquiry by men of knowledge who possess authority in their fields (p. 17). In this sense, for Phenix, the 'realms of meaning' determine scope and these are socially determined in his broad framework schema for a general curriculum (p. 18). Phenix (1964) would also argue that the essential character of whole fields of knowledge should be brought out by what he calls 'key concepts', and thus for Phenix emphasis looms strongly in curricular design.

Wheeler (1967) sees scope related to the aims and goals (p. 145), and should include provision for the establishment of patterns of behaviour to include the widest possible range of experiences. In viewing scope as a vital consideration in selection, the identification of fundamentals of subject matter in terms of universals, abstractions and specifics are important for Wheeler (p. 215). In other words, relationships and principles are more important than facts, and applying what is learned is more important than merely learning it.

Taba (1962) suggests that each pattern of curriculum adopts a certain idea of scope because it adopts certain centres of organisation (p. 382). In effect, decisions made regarding the centre of focus such as a theme or a unitary approach through modules, determines the way in which the scope of the entire curriculum will be considered. In this context, if the basic modular units are organised in terms of subjects and topics, the coverage of the content becomes the main way of determining the scope. In effect, if basic ideas and concepts become criteria for scope, they do so because they are important centres for organising units of the curriculum, and to this extent reflect comprehensive application to the various areas of knowledge and their interrelationships.

A further useful indicator for determining the broad scope of a programme in relationship to relevance for the learners is to identify content that the student must know, content that the student should know and lastly content that the student could know. These three considerations are important for determining priorities and focal emphasis.

If scope means identifying what has to be covered and learned in terms of subjects, topics, objectives and processes, fundamental decisions rest on certain value considerations of what is worthwhile, or in Hirst's analysis (1975), what is *most* worthwhile. Scope is also related to this value factor often through themes or 'core' threads in the curriculum which can attempt to develop central worthwhile factors or indicate emphasis.

Within a content framework, themes or core elements may serve as 'organising centres' in the operational sense and usually involve questions related to teaching approach, variety and form of learning experiences, assessment of learners in terms of interests, needs (needs assessment), instructional materials and available educational technology.

In this sense, scope is concerned not just with a consideration of content in terms of main ideals and factual information and their relationship within the curricular framework, but also with the necessary treatments or learning experience arrangements which are design factors themselves related to the processing of the content. In addition to content and process problems, scope may well have to take account of traditions, what has preceded the new curriculum, what has stood the test of time before and is deemed by tradition to be valuable and worthwhile. Finally, certain external constraints extrinsic to the curriculum may be applied by external agencies such as professional bodies and statutory bodies, which act to mediate and produce scope determinants that the planners are forced to give evidence to. On the other hand, external influence can be sought such as expert opinion on particular disciplines or subject fields, or from research and experimentation. Also, practical applications such as 'task-analysis', job-analysis or systems evaluation can be used which will help to determine scope.

Sequence and Continuity

Sequence concerns the order in which content and processes are presented to the learner, and the main concern is with the development of what is thought to be the correct sequence of tasks that will systematically yield predictable forms of student behaviour. Sequence involves the spatial relationship of content and processes. Order of difficulty is often seen as fundamental, and in almost any sequence there is a noticeable attempt to move from simple to complex, from concrete to abstract and from the immediate to the wider and more remote.

The sequence of design is strongly related to the 'when' criteria and to questions of duration (the 'how long?' aspect). Thus timing and length of units and lessons are important, as is the principle that information and learning experiences be presented at the time they are of greatest use to the students. Similarly there are considerations of logic. For instance, Taba (1962, p. 81) would use the 'logic of the content' to pursue those questions that represent important aspects of rational pattern. Gagné (1965) would consider the prerequisite knowledge required, and move from the known to the unknown, from the concrete to the abstract generalisations and from universals to specifics. Within this psychological approach there is an incremental logic as well as a logic related to the nature of the content and the student's ability to come to terms with it.

Integration

Two aspects of integration are useful considerations for designing curricular structures: (i) the mechanical structure of integration which to some extent follows on from scope and sequence, and (ii) content integration. In considering the mechanics of structure, Tyler (1950) has stressed the ideas of continuity, sequence and integration. For Tyler, continuity is the vertical reiteration of elements. Sequence involves building on previous experience but going more broadly and deeply, and integration is the horizontal relationships of the curriculum experience. Schrader (1972) sees continuity as the number of consecutive tasks in which a given theme is present. Anderson (1971) uses the term commonality, which he uses to represent 'contiguous' units with matching elements. Contiguous units with unmatched elements are termed progressive (or progression) by the same author. Briggs (1967) considers vertical structure as a dependence of each vertically ordered element on the one immediately preceding and views hierarchical structure as the teaching of component skills in association with more complex ones. He sees flat structures as independent elements. Bruner (1960) suggests the idea of spiralling in which learning and content reappear in more complex forms as part of a given theme. Gagné (1965) suggests hierarchical arrangements, and Johnson, M. (1967) a structure of intended learning outcomes. Postner (1974) sees curriculum structurally conceptualised at different levels of generality depending on whether micro- or macro-elements are involved. In this sense he sees micro-elements as such things as individual intended learnings, performances and capabilities, and sees macro-elements (categories of micro-elements) as such items as lesson, unit, course or programme. The macro-elements are usually described in syllabi, curriculum guides and programme sequences. Bernstein (1971) puts forward a classification as an approach to areas of study. As a classification, however, the approach is not strictly taxonomic, for Bernstein refers not to what is classified but to the relationship between contents. Thus, the approach is within the mechanism of structure. Where classification is strong, contents are well insulated from each other by strong boundaries. Where classification is weak there is reduced insulation between contents, for the boundaries between contents are weak or blurred.

Taba (1962, p. 36) and Wheeler (1967, p. 249) both suggest the usefulness of organising centres for integrative purposes. Taba sees 'key ideas' or the dimension of topics as centres for organising content and learning experiences. Phenix (1964, p. 238) suggests a hierarchy of concepts that can be constructed for each of his six fields or realms by which they serve to guide the teacher in the instructional task. Goodland and Richter (1963) suggests that topics, problems, units of work or resource units are the organising elements of an organising centre. Bloom (1958) suggests integrative threads by which learning experiences are related and gives criteria for selecting, developing and using them by using major topics, ideas and theories in a single subject field, or methods of thought and work and types of inquiry to relate diverse content and different types of problems (p. 85).

Wheeler (1967, p. 262) stresses the need to have criteria of suitable organisation that keep in focus both the learning experiences, the content and its nature by way of learning outcomes. In this sense, for Wheeler, the organising centres will in general be the basic core or focussing ideas that link the parallel sequences of content and developmental activities. Concentration on outcomes provides guidelines for selecting the specific details of content so that organising centres attempt to cater for achievement of outcomes by matching learning activities and subject matter.

(vi) Integration and the Nursing Curriculum

The focus of integration in the nursing curriculum must initially concentrate on structuring, ordering and sequencing content by seeking to unify nursing practice and nursing theory. The focus must also seek to organise the curriculum so that the learner is assisted in securing, assimilating and applying specific contents, concepts and principles. Nursing 'practice' and nursing 'theory' must in this sense be seen as aspects of knowledge that are holistic and interdependent. The intent of this curricular approach is to promote an awareness of the wholeness or unity of the discipline of nursing. In this context it is necessary to include interlocking courses or content from varied subject areas that are antecedent to nursing, as well as courses dealing with specific nursing subject areas.

A common assumption about integration is that it occurs within the individual and that this internalised integration should be a major aim in education. If this is the case the integration within a curriculum can be looked at in terms of it being a process or a series of operations or functions, which produce the essential balance to bring about unity. As such, the components are related in such a way as to form a functional whole, a completeness or entirety and the curriculum structure, methods and experiences should be designed to promote and support this idea of internalised integration. Knudsen (1937) designated a type of interaction between parts within the individual and also between the individual and his environment.

Heidergerken (1955) and Johansen (1951) refer to integration as a form of unification which also applies to learning methods and to content. Styles (1976) discusses integration in terms of relationships among the knowledge, skills and values learned. Although there seems to be a general acceptance of wholeness as the intent of integration, there are considerable differences of opinion regarding where the focus of integration should be.

Parker (1894) and Torres (1974) apply the wholeness intent of integration primarily to subject matter, while Henry (1958) and Hopkins (1935) focus on integration by the learner. Members of the National League of Nursing have applied the idea of integration to both subject matter and to the learner. Weitzel (1980), in considering a philosophical base for the integrated nursing curriculum, also focuses on the wholeness intent of integration which is defined as including the plan and means for achieving learning goals (p. 23). Welch and Slagle (1980) also view integration as a way of organising the curriculum to assist the learner in analysing and applying the relationship of content, concepts and principles in their nursing practice. They also stress the internalisation of knowledge by the learner. Certainly there is too often an assumption that the student can absorb differentiated knowledge and, at the same time, integrate this knowledge. Welch and Slagle (*ibid*., p. 39) believe that the 'nursing process' as an overall conceptual approach should be used to provide the integrating structure for the curriculum in nursing.

It seems that intentions to integrate nursing knowledge can be handled in a variety of ways. Core curricula, correlated curricula and broad conceptual approaches are common in the United States of America and it does appear that the trend has been one in which facts are learned, knowledge integrated, and knowledge generalised using a medical curricular model. The emerging trend since the late 1970s has been through an increasingly distinctive nursing model operationalised by considering the characteristics of the nursing process. In this particular trend it has been essential for the curriculum designers to identify the order, structure, scope and depth of nursing content to facilitate student learning and not just to integrate the nursing content.

If wholeness as unity is the major intent of an integrated nursing curriculum and if the nursing process is increasingly accepted as a major referent for securing effective integration, many other elements such as objectives, the conceptual framework, learning experience and evaluation modes must be taken into account. The referents of wholeness must also include: man, as a learner and as a patient or client; society, including the family, cultures and social institutions; health, as it affects the individual and society; nursing, as a discipline and a process; and learning, as a product and a process. In essence, beliefs about man, society, health, nursing and learning would be common referents for integrative themes in the nursing curriculum.

(vii) Teaching and Learning Activities

The basic design of a curriculum cannot be realistically considered without the evidence provided by educational psychologists about learning and instruction. Consequently, how to facilitate learning in a planned environment has been a major concern and is reflected in the work of Anderson (1967), Frase (1975), Gagné and Rowher (1969), Glaser and Resnick (1970) and McKeachie (1974). Instruction throughout these authors' writings is seen as a phenomenon that involves both planning of the learning environment and the appropriate teaching techniques to bring about instructional events. The design specification must, therefore, include the intentions for dealing with these instructional events in some purposeful way that will ensure that the learning desired is more likely to occur. In other words, a clear specification of instructional intent has to be made which indicates the modes of teacher-learner activities in relationship to specific content and objectives.

A considerable wealth of learning and instructional evidence has been developed over the years and is relevant to the application of learning principles to instructional events. Bruner (1971) stresses the need for structured learning and instruction, Gagné (1965) favours sequenced instructional events, and Bloom (1976) has demonstrated the value of systematic planning as a variable that produces higher achievement levels. Fuller (1969) and Treffinger (1977) want sequence of content to be related to sequence in instruction. Gagné (1965) is also concerned with design factors in which learning is equated with a hierarchical structure of events to produce behavioural performance changes.

Schwab (1969) stresses inquiry strategies in which the method of inquiry is based on the syntax of the subject content. Gagné and White (1978) see variety of learning enhancing understanding and promoting the transfer of learning. Ausubel (1967) relates the learning at hand to the learner's own cognitive structures and stresses the use of concept learning and of advance organisers to stimulate recall of previously learned material. Klix (1971) stresses the use of concepts, Elshout and Elshout (1969) creative reasoning, and Dirkzwager (1974) logical problem solving. Carol (1963) and Glaser (1967) favour individual learning approaches, while Alpern (1966), Hamilton (1967) and Keller (1978) have all used self-directed learning approaches involving self-pacing which have been found to improve performance on a variety of courses.

A wide variety of possible approaches is available and although there is no totally coherent set of explanations to guide the use of instructional methods, there is sufficient range for sensitive choices to be made. The choices of method must relate to attempts to produce the best kinds of learning experiences which are most likely to meet the objectives of the course. The planning exercise in respect of teaching arrangements should be concerned with structuring a series of learning outcomes by taking into account the conceptual structure of the content, possible ways of retrieving and dealing with information and optimising the transfer of learning. The conceptual framework of the course must also be carefully considered so that learning experiences can be arranged in a sequential order and provision be made for learning to proceed from known to unknown, from concrete to abstract, and from operational thought to generalisations.

The learning experiences provided in the course should be so arranged that a variety of behaviours and skills are developed and the extension of attitudes and feelings is made possible. In this respect the learning experiences chosen for the course should provide for multiple kinds of learning, such as inquiry, problem-solving and experimentation, both collaboratively and independently. If by instruction we mean deliberate interventions in the learning process of an individual learner, then the interventions must be planned as sequences and interrelated events, not as chance occurrences. Thus developing motivation, directing attention to objectives, guiding learning, enhancing retention, promoting transfer, developing performance and providing feedback are all aspects of the structured interventions in learning that we call instruction.

(viii) Evaluation

It is not proposed in this section to give an extensive review of the literature and curricular evaluative thinking which are currently influencing curriculum; space alone will not permit this. What is intended is to relate the importance of evaluation to the design structure of the nursing curriculum. Curriculum evaluation can be characterised in a variety of ways depending on the purpose of the evaluation and who is making the evaluation. As such the nature of evaluation can range from a very comprehensive analysis to a very sharp focus on a single element of the curriculum. Similarly many people can be involved in evaluation, ranging from educator, administrator and curricular specialist to employer and consumer. Evaluation should be recognised as an integral part of all the phases of the curriculum and should operate as a continuous process. It will involve the systematic collection and use of data so that judgements can be made throughout the development and operationalisation of the curriculum. It should involve more than just testing and the measurement of student learning outcomes; indeed, any aspect and often most aspects of a course can be evaluated.

Two major forms of evaluation may be helpful in the evaluation of the nursing curriculum. These are known as formative evaluation and summative evaluation respectively, as broadly characterised by Scriven (1967). Formative evaluation occurs while the curriculum is being implemented and is usually done at recurring intervals so that feedback can be provided related to operational problems. The operational problems within the programme are the actual curricular events such as goal achievements, the effects of the instructional activities and the nature and consequences of learning experiences and outcomes. In these instances the evaluation focuses on the provisions, procedures and processes within the curriculum. Summative evaluation is more concerned with the overall influences and consequences of quality control and the effectiveness of the curriculum over a long period of time. In this respect, identifying desirable qualitative factors and standards is important and maintaining quality and detecting deterioration in quality are important inclusions for the evaluative procedures.

From a planning point of view it is essential to have a curricular evaluative framework or a scheme that is both systematic and comprehensive. Finch and Bjorkquist (1977) suggest a scheme of four elements of evaluation which are presented as: (1) context evaluation, (2) input evaluation, (3) process evaluation, and (4) product evaluation. Shufflebeam (1969) also proposed context, input, process and product (CIPP).

(1) Context Evaluation

The context evaluation is concerned with what type of curriculum should be offered and what goals and objectives should be used and relate to the curriculum when it is being initiated and structured. Questions are related to the definition and description of the environment in which the curriculum will be offered and to some extent set the actual parameters or extent of the curriculum. Identification is made of whom the curriculum will serve, what content will be included, what goals and objectives the curriculum should have and use. Data can be derived from the School of Nursing, the students and consumers and by student participation in the evaluation of courses. Observations are made of intended and unintended achievement of objectives and needs assessment and task analysis are required in context evaluation. By its nature, context evaluation is mostly subjective and speculative, particularly with respect to content, which has to be guided by the available models of nursing and the changing nature of social health requirements.

(2) Input Evaluation

This focuses on resources and strategies for decision-making. Reasons are required for the selection of particular resources and making proper use of them. Relevant questions include: What curricular materials are most suitable for teachers and learners? What educational resources are best for a particular educational setting? How might learning and instructional events best be implemented? In these instances consideration will be given to things such as space, equipment, materials and support services in both the school and the clinical experiences in the hospitals and the community. Reports and observations will be taken from involved persons. Informal and formal feedback through questionnaires, interviews or discussions will be made with nurse teachers, students and clinical nursing staff in hospital and community. Observations will be made on the influence upon and provisions for student learning. Procedures such as teacher-learner strategies and policies for their curricular implementation will be analysed by direct observation and reports made available. Formal and informal discussions involving staff and student bodies and school committees will be sources for much of the data, as well as direct observations of student responses and attitudes to curriculum procedure. Evidence of student learning and comparison of student attitudes to achievement of objectives would be other valuable data sources. Data gathering for input evaluation will range from simple to complex, using instruments with varying degrees of objectivity.

(3) Process Evaluation

This deals directly with the operation of the curriculum and is in the traditional sense what many people think of as being evaluation itself. This element of evaluation is focused on the instructional and learning events. It seeks to find out how well the learners are performing and to examine the effectiveness and quality of the instruction and those involved in its arrangements. It also attempts to find the degree of student satisfaction and which if any of the curricular components are ineffective or deficient. Inevitably the interaction between students and teachers and subject matter are under scrutiny. Evidence of student learning is sought from direct observations and reports from involved persons. Data related to input from students and teaching staff regarding their perceptions of the curriculum process are considered. Observation of classroom interaction and evidence of changes in attitudes or values will be important considerations. Comparisons of student attitudes to achievement of objectives are also essential. Methods used in process evaluation are various and include teacher behaviour measures, teaching rating measures, standard achievement measures, teacher constructed tests, clinical nursing performance tests, pre- and post-modular tests, and the like.

(4) Product Evaluation

Product evaluation takes place typically 'in the field' with information being gathered from sources such as employers, supervisors and former students in the occupational context.

Wentling and Lawson (1975) view the elements of product evaluation as important, because process evaluation deals only with short-term effects. Product evaluation looks at the mobility of former students and seeks to find out how satisfied they are with post-course and occupational achievements. This covers job specification, job satisfaction and skills associated with the job that have been influenced by the curriculum. Employer views of the performance of former students are important in determining how adequate the curriculum is for preparing individuals for the job. In nursing the product evaluation would appraise the newly registered nurse and his/her performance in the work setting. Data could be achieved through reports from involved persons. Questionnaires sent to newly registered nurses one year following registration could determine attainment of course objectives. Direct observations could be made on newly qualified nurses of intended and unintended results through the use of rating scales, systematic observation and unstructured observation. Comparison of student entrance characteristics, attitudes, perception, motivation, and behaviour with characteristics upon qualification could be made as evidence of student learning.

The above assumptions are based on the Phi Delta Kappa Committee Model, with which Shufflebeam (1969) is closely associated. It is essentially a decision-making model or a decision-oriented model and there appears to be considerable systematic benefit to be gained from its use in nursing courses where a rational evaluation approach is required. The context evaluation assesses objectives and target populations (type of student). The input evaluation determines the best use of resources and how they can be used to reach the goals. The process evaluation views the actual course operations and the logistics of implementation. Product evaluation examines whether objectives have been achieved. All four evaluation elements affect decisions concerning the ultimate degree of success of the curriculum.

4 A CURRICULUM MODEL FOR NURSING

(i) Introduction

The nursing curriculum model proposed in this book is based on a dual use of existing models, (i) the nursing process and (ii) the curriculum process. It is my intention to inter-relate the central paradigms of each of these models to produce a nursing curriculum model from which nursing courses can be rationally planned, implemented and evaluated. The nursing process which is relatively new to nursing in the United Kingdom and the curriculum process which is increasingly being used in general education are strikingly similar both structurally and functionally. Both have a dynamic nature and represent organisational modes of thinking about nursing and education. Both processes represent the interactive nature of events between individuals in the sense that nursing is an interaction between nurse and patient, and the curriculum in the instructional sense is an interaction between teacher and learner. Both the nursing process and the curriculum process have similar elements in their structures and both can operate as cyclic and continuously adjusting mechanisms (see Figure 1). Both have a relatively simple logic in approach which can be identified in the phase-by-phase sequence in the planning and development involved. Both processes use objectives, planning strategies, evaluation procedures and a methodology developed as technologies.

Nurses assess patients and plan their care and evaluate this care through the nursing process, and in doing so create nursing interventions or 'nursing events'. Teachers assess their students, plan teaching, implement teaching and learning interventions and in doing so create 'instructional events' which are evaluated for effectiveness. Nurse teachers have to be able to operate within both these processes and students of nursing are exposed to both of these processes.

Although strikingly similar in their overall structure, there are differences in the individual events which make up the four phases in each model. Both processes have a simple logic based on objective thinking rather than complex theoretical assumptions. This apparent simplicity should be attractive to both nurses and nurse teachers, not because either are simplistic in their thinking (for they are not) but because the simple rational approach has a much more realistic chance of being used in the day-to-day turmoil of the nursing environment and nursing educational contexts.

Figure 1: The Relationship of the Curriculum Process's Four Major Elements to the Nursing Process as a Cyclical Activity.

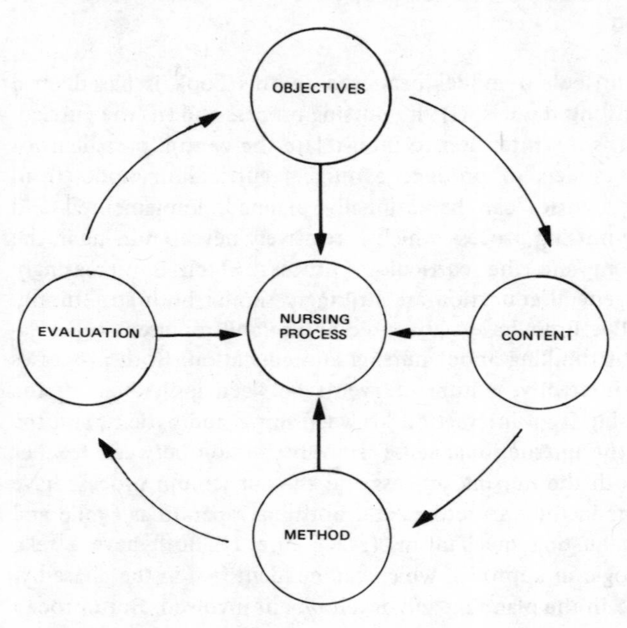

In the first phase of each process there is an implicit concern to identify intentions. The first phase of the nursing process is directed at the assessment of the patient to identify his problems and needs, help him adapt to his immediate problems and decide his potentiality for restoration to a state of health. From the assessment of the patient, data are collected and analysed from which the objectives of the intended nursing care are proposed as nursing intentions. In this way the anticipated nursing outcomes are specified as clear intentions that are called the nursing objectives.

The corresponding first phase in the curriculum process is concerned with identifying the learning needs of the student, his potential learning problems, and specifying the forms of learning performance that are required in order to attain and develop specific knowledge and skills. The learning outcomes are specified as clear intentions that are known as learning objectives. In the nursing process the nursing intentions are used to produce nursing events which effect gains towards a predetermined outcome – health. The curriculum intentions are used to produce instructional events which effect gains in the student to a predetermined outcome – nursing education.

The second phase of the nursing process is concerned with determining the nature of the nursing events and using a planning structure for the organisation of the nursing interventions in order to secure achievements of the prescribed nursing objectives. The second phase of the curriculum process is concerned with determining the content to be learned and the relationships of the particular knowledge and skills within a particular set of sequences over a particular range of material in order to achieve the prescribed learning objectives.

The third phase of the nursing process is directed at implementing the planned nursing events or the delivery of nursing care to the patient, and it is within this phase that the technologies of nursing are identified, selected and used. The third phase of the curriculum process is directed at implementing the planned instructional events or the provision of learning experiences for the student, and it is within this phase that the methods as technologies of instruction are identified, selected and used. In both instances the technologies of nursing and teaching are complementary to the creative ability of the nurse and teacher in the sense that they are both creative forms of personal service.

The final phase of both processes is concerned with evaluation. In the nursing process, evaluation is concerned with judging the value or worth and the effectiveness of the nursing event including the quality of care and the extent to which the nursing objectives have been achieved. In the curriculum process, evaluation is concerned with judging the value or worth of the instructional event, the effectiveness and quality of the learning experience and the extent to which the learning objectives have been achieved.

Both processes are concerned with personal and individual development in health on the one hand and education on the other. The nursing process is essentially designed to both individualise and personalise the nursing events in patient care. Similarly, the curriculum process can be used to both individualise and personalise the instructional events and the learning experiences within nursing education to a much greater extent than has been the case in the past. In both contexts, nursing can be made more effective as an individual process and the learning of nursing care can make greater use of individualised learning (though not exclusively) through the use of the curriculum process.

(ii) The Nursing Curriculum Model

My suggestion is the combination of the nursing process model and the curriculum process model (see Figures 1 and 2) to produce a nursing curriculum model. Such a combination of models with the inclusion of the correct antecedent nursing knowledge and specific nursing knowledge itself dervied mainly from on-going research, can be the framework for nursing curriculum development. The combination of the nursing process model and the curriculum process model can be effectively used in nursing curriculum development and will be valuable in giving clearer identification of what should be taught and direction to how it should be taught by giving effective organisational structure to the curriculum.

Figure 2: The Relationship of the Four Phases of the Curriculum Process to the Four Phases of the Nursing Process. The outer circle of activity, the curriculum processes (objectives, content, methods and evaluation), are seen in relationship to each of the four phases of the nursing process which are represented as the inner circle of activity.

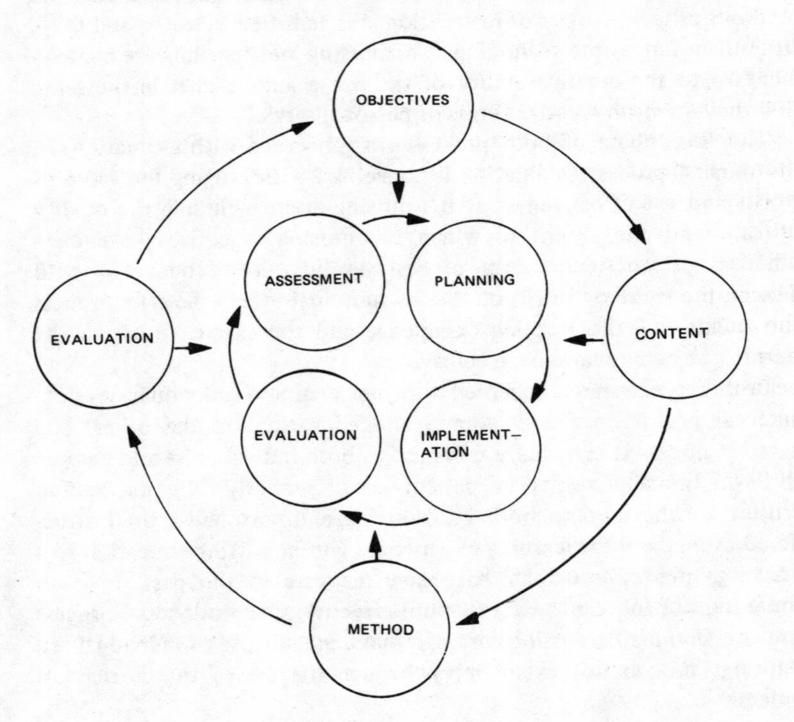

The nursing curriculum, whether it be in courses, units or modules, can be effectively organised around the four phases of the nursing process using their major concepts (assessment, planning, implementation and evaluation) as organising and integrating curricular themes. The model can also be used as an organising framework for theoretical assumptions about nursing derived from the various models of nursing which have been reviewed in the preceding chapters. The conceptual thinking within these models can be accommodated into the four phases of the nursing process to allow an eclectic use of currently developing nursing knowledge. Similarly, the antecedents of nursing knowledge (the elements of biological and behavioural sciences) can also be incorporated into the four phases of the nursing process and made operational within the nursing curriculum by using the curriculum process. The approximation of four distinct but potentially interrelating areas thus form the nursing curriculum model and are respectively (i) antecedent nursing knowledge, (ii) specific nursing knowledge, (iii) the nursing process, and (iv) the curriculum process. The model and its four relationships can be viewed as represented in Figure 3.

Although the major purpose of the proposed model is to rationalise the planning and operation of the nursing curriculum and not necessarily to specify distinct detailed content, it is necessary to give some indication of the broad areas of content to which the nursing process and the curriculum process can relate in terms of broad themes. Two such broad themes inherent within the model are (i) the antecedents of nursing knowledge, and (ii) specific nursing knowledge. I use the term nursing knowledge to include the technical, behavioural and intellectual abilities required to make effective nursing interactions with patients. The term antecedent nursing knowledge is used in this context to mean the technical, behavioural and intellectual abilities required to form the bases of nursing knowledge which are derived from the biological and behavioural sciences. The possession of such abilities is necessarily antecedent to nursing knowledge itself.

Antecedent Nursing Knowledge

Within the model proposed, antecedent nursing knowledge is seen to be concerned with the study of the living person as a whole and should draw on principles and laws that govern life processes, well-being and the optimum functioning of human beings whether sick or well. In this respect, biologically derived principles of nursing care are seen to be important prerequisites and are directed to the physical incapacity of patients emphasising the sickness and the pathology involved.

Figure 3: The Nursing Curriculum Model

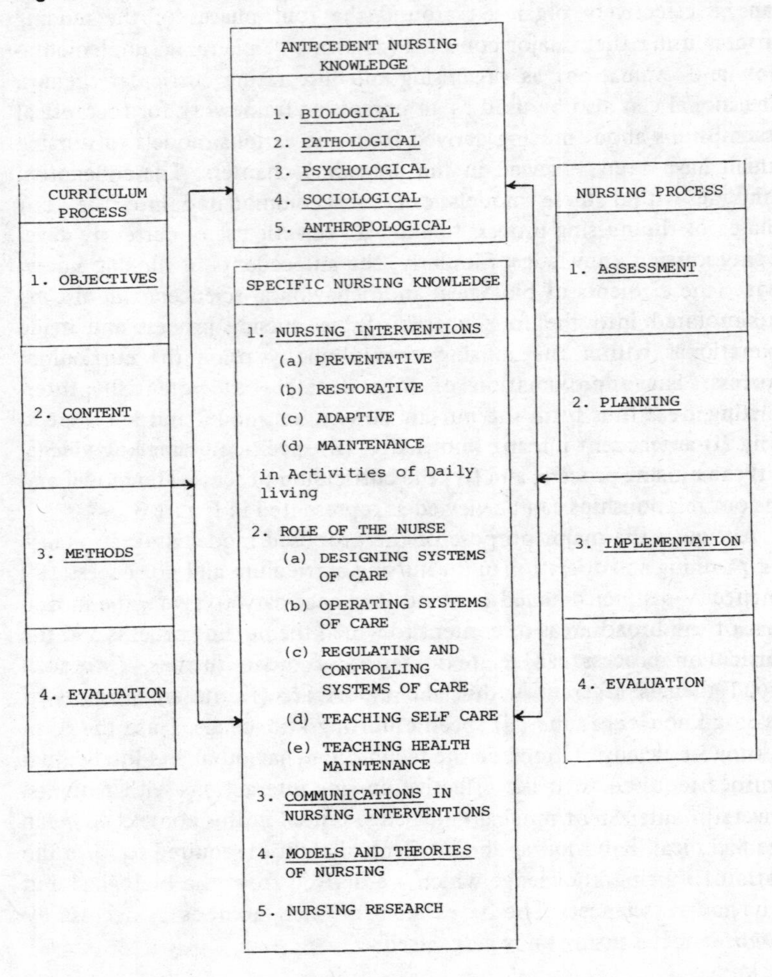

Although there is a strong lobby within the nursing establishment to reject the disease element of the medical model, nursing cannot ignore the fact that patients are suffering from diseases, and the student of nursing must be familiar at least to some extent with their cause and effect in the biopathological sense, in order to understand the physical problems of the patient which are external manifestations of the disease. Physiological disturbances in the patient are a result or cause of the disease process and they are important elements in the consideration of nursing care strategies for individual patients. It is in this particular sense that biopathological considerations are antecedent to specific nursing knowledge.

Antecedent nursing knowledge is also concerned with the various patterns and form of human behaviour with respect to individuals, groups and society as a whole. It is therefore essential that specific nursing knowledge draws from psychology, sociology and elements of anthropology to produce psychologically, sociologically and anthropologically derived principles of nursing care. In this respect the ideas of the person as a whole, his interaction with other individuals and the ways in which social, cultural and institutional arrangements create problems and disease are important antecedents to specific nursing knowledge. It is my suggestion therefore that biology, pathology, psychology, sociology and anthropology are the most suitable disciplines from which the broad fields of antecedent nursing knowledge can be formed to produce the basic knowledge elements required by the nurse to create specific nursing skills and abilities, that can be used in the organisational contexts of the nursing process.

The Biological Basis of Nursing Practice. This is an important antecedent for nursing knowledge and the nursing curriculum should provide a basic theoretical and practical study which should include appropriate elements of histology, biochemistry, embryology, anatomy and physiology. The essential intention of the curriculum designer when organising biological content for nurses should be the development in the student of knowledge, skills, attitudes and values derived from a study of the human body that will assist the nurse to develop excellence in the delivery of nursing care to patients. Developing within the student the capacity to understand the fundamental principles of human biology in relation to deepening and broadening her understanding of the human body in health and disease is a priority for creative nursing care. It is *a priori* to developing and extending the student's ability to use biological knowledge in effectively assessing, planning, implementing and evaluating nursing care for individual patients.

The following general objectives for the biological basis of the curriculum for nurses would be useful considerations for the curriculum maker and the curriculum user:

(1) The student should have knowledge of those aspects of the biological sciences which are relevant to a definition of the optimum conditions for the promotion of health, prevention of

disease, management of illness and delivery of nursing care.

(2) The student should be able to identify and use those biological principles which will enable her to develop methods of assessment of patients and promote the development of alternative innovative methods in the planning, implementation and evaluation of nursing care.

(3) The student should also have appropriate knowledge of those biological principles which will enable her to perform nursing care safely and to the appropriate standard.

(4) The student should have knowledge of appropriate published research in the biological sciences which is relevant to nursing practice, and she should be able to demonstrate that she can incorporate where appropriate research findings in the assessment of patients and in the planning, implementation and evaluation of nursing care.

The Social and Psychological Basis of Nursing Practice. Collectively the behavioural sciences are essential knowledge areas for consideration in the development of a curriculum for nurses. Appropriate eclectic use of the fields of knowledge which concern themselves with human behaviour, whether individual or group, social systems or cultures, and cultural differences, is required. These fields are previously neglected areas of study for the majority of nurses and few curricular attempts in the past have really exploited the enormous potential that these fields of study have in the education of nurses and the humanising of the care of the sick. The curriculum maker and the curriculum user must give major consideration to these important nursing antecedents. The content of the nursing curriculum must take a much more serious account both in width and depth of a theoretical and practical study of social behaviour from which the fundamental principles can be applied to the nursing care of patients. Similarly and in parallel a theoretical and practical study of human psychological development and behaviour must be used from which fundamental principles can be applied to the nursing care of individual patients. Both social and psychological inputs should be structured and operationalised to develop in the student, knowledge, skills, attitudes and values that can be applied to the nursing of patients to give excellence in care.

The following general objectives for the social and psychological basis of nursing practice should be considered:

(1) The student should have the knowledge and ability to apply the

concepts employed in behavioural science to nursing care.

(2) The student should be able to relate practical applications of nursing care to behavioural science inputs.

(3) The student should be able to identify and use those behavioural science considerations which will be relevant to specific health care and nursing contexts.

(4) The student should be able to make critical evaluation of appropriate behavioural science research for application to nursing care.

The nursing curriculum should allow for the student to gain knowledge of those aspects of behavioural science upon which modern nursing practice may be based. This should be done in such a way that the student is able to consider behavioural science as a major contribution to the investigation and improvement of nursing care.

Anthropology as an Input to Basic Nursing Knowledge. Contemporary cross-cultural and ethological studies of human behaviour are increasingly seen as relevant knowledge for study by nurses. The cultural differences which exist in most advanced civilised societies have profound effects on the health care systems within these societies. Traditional and holistic healing, its relevance to health issues in communities, and the cultural differences in notions of health and sickness, disease and cure, are major influencing factors on the way in which health care is perceived and organised.

The importance of cultural differences for nurses and nursing has been admirably demonstrated in Leininger's (1978) text. The relevance of cross-cultural study and the validity of techniques to investigate domestic health issues are concisely dealt with to present an excellent overview of anthropological relevance. The social culture in which the student of nursing will learn nursing and later practise nursing as a professional influences her own personal development and her nursing practice. The student needs to learn the importance and value of customs, habits and mores, as a basis for effective cultural and social relations in nursing care activities with patients.

Equally important for the student in the understanding of nursing as a professional health care activity are the cultural determinants seen in the evolution of nursing as an occupational group. The notion of how nurses perceive themselves and how they are perceived by other health care groups is an important area of cultural analysis which can help the nurse play a more positive role as a collaborative health care worker. Such study can help nurses to a deeper understanding of individual and collective health care behaviour, and with an imaginative curricular application form part of the necessary antecedent knowledge for nursing.

The following general objectives for anthropological elements relative to a social studies input to the basis of nursing practice are offered as useful considerations for the curriculum. The student should be able to:

(1) Discuss cultural determinants in the evolution of nursing and analyse the relationships between nursing and other health care groups and professions.
(2) Determine cultural differences in the social structures of the hospital and other health care contexts.
(3) Explain cultural transmission within the general process of socialisation.
(4) Critically analyse the notion of culture and the elements which constitute one.
(5) Identify and specify cultural differences in notions of health, sickness, disease and cure.
(6) Analyse and determine the relevance and validity of cross-cultural studies in appropriate nursing care contexts.

The Pathological Basis of Nursing Practice. Much emphasis has recently been directed at 'debunking' the so-called 'medical model' and the notion of disease as an area of study for nurses has come under persistent attack. Whilst the critics of disease-oriented nursing curricula have idealistic motives underpinning the popular current movement toward a 'nursing model', it would be totally illogical to expect modern professional nurses to organise and effectively deliver nursing care to patients without some knowledge of the underlying disease processes that cause their patients to be sick. To include within the curriculum less detailed pathology than that which is included in syllabi for comparable paramedical professional groups would be seriously disadvantaging the nurse's position within the health care team.

It is a matter of course of determining what are the most appropriate aspects of disease nurses should know and of securing relevant application to the art and science of nursing. In this sense a pathological element is a vital antecedent of nursing practice. Whilst it must be seen that nursing *per se* should dominate the nursing curriculum as the specific area of knowledge, and given that health care must be as important as illness care, there must be a contribution to nursing knowledge from human biological disorder.

How much nurses need to study the biological disorder as a disease response within the patient must be determined by the circumstances of the day in terms of the maladies that dominate in sickness and disease in society. To divorce disease as an appropriate area of study from nursing would be as unrealistic as current attempts to divorce nursing and doctoring as complementary and intersupporting activities. The following general objectives for the pathological basis of nursing practice are offered as useful considerations for the curriculum. The student:

(1) Should have knowledge of those aspects of pathology which are relevant to a definition of the optimum conditions for the management of illness and the delivery of nursing care.
(2) Should have appropriate knowledge of those pathological principles which will enable her effectively to perform preventative, restorative, adaptive and maintenance nursing interventions, safely and to a desired standard.
(3) Should be able to use those pathological principles which will enable her to develop methods of assessment of patients, and promote the development of alternative innovative methods in the planning, implementation and evaluation of nursing care.
(4) Should be able to identify and use those pathological principles which will enable her to work effectively in collaboration with medical, paramedical and other health care workers.

Nursing Knowledge (Specific)

Specific nursing knowledge is concerned with the functional activity of the nurse and includes her role and the nursing events that are directed to the individual patient. The nursing care concerns the patient's activities of daily living, and the events that make up that care in an individualised and personalised way are termed nursing interventions.

Nursing interventions are the skilled application of technical, behavioural and intellectual abilities that form the nursing care of the patient. The nursing interventions are designed, operated and regulated through the use of the nursing process and in such a way that the conditions of nursing care are controlled and rationally organised.

The nursing interventions are preventative, restorative or adaptive, or contain elements of all three. When nursing interventions are preventative the nursing events are designed to inhibit effects detrimental to the patient's health. When nursing interventions are restorative the nursing events are those that return the patient's functioning to the normal or optimal level. When the nursing interventions are adaptive the nursing events are designed to adapt the patient within certain limits with respect to the activities of daily living but below full health capacity. Within prevention, restoration and adaption, the nurse functions by assisting, enabling and teaching the patient to perform and maintain daily living activities.

The functional activities of nursing therefore must be the central frame of reference for the specific knowledge that constitutes nursing itself as a unique form of health care. The functional activities of nursing in this respect (what nurses do and how they do it) must be the central content of the nursing curriculum and may be represented in the following ten perspectives;

(1) Preventative nursing interventions in the activities of daily living.
(2) Restorative nursing interventions in the activities of daily living.
(3) Adaptive nursing interventions in the activities of daily living.
(4) Maintenance nursing interventions in the activities of daily living.
(5) Communication and nursing interactions in nursing interventions.
(6) The role and function of the nurse in designing processes and systems of nursing care for individuals and groups.
(7) The role and function of the nurse in operating processes and systems of nursing care for individuals and groups.
(8) The role and function of the nurse in regulating and controlling processes and systems of nursing care for individuals and groups.
(9) The role and function of the nurse in teaching individuals and groups to perform and maintain self-care in the activities of daily living.
(10) The role and function of the nurse in teaching individuals and groups to prevent deviations in health.

Within these ten perspectives the function of nurses and nursing are the dominant *modus operandi* for the nursing curriculum, with emphasis on the learner nurses being educated to become safe practitioners and to fill adequately the roles they must perform in a changing world of nursing.

Consideration of specific nursing as a knowledge area must place curricular emphasis on enabling the student to master the appropriate nursing knowledge and skills to solve the problems of patients with respect to nursing care. To make effective use of the nursing process as a systematic method of organising and managing nursing care the nurse must possess a range of technical nursing skills which are appropriate to the specific nursing care events which the patient receives in the overall care provided.

The development of technical nursing skills in the student and ability to use procedures and methods that have utility for providing solutions to patient problems should be a major focus of specific nursing knowledge in the curriculum. These techniques or basic fundamental nursing methods (those previously known as basic nursing care skills), which constitute the personal aspects of patient care, have to be presented, conceptualised and taught within patient-problem centred contexts. Emphasis has to be directed at the individual and personalised approaches to patient care which provide for basic human needs or functions and help people with their daily activities of living.

Henderson (1978) clearly conceptualises the nature of the curricular content for nurses when she argues that the student should be given the opportunity to help patients attain a high state of wellness, prevent disease, achieve independence after illness, cope with handicap, or accept death (p. 126). The competence needed within technical nursing ability to do this will depend considerably on exposing the student to a wide range of nursing problems requiring a more diversified exercise of professional competence than has been the case in the past.

It is desirable for the student both to experience and to participate in a wide range of care settings, including the patient's home, clinics, hospitals, nursing homes, schools and industrial settings. Such experience should allow the student to accommodate a comprehensive overview of the health care problems in society. Teaching the basic principles of nursing care and developing the technical nursing skills in a student are, on their own, not enough. The skills acquired by the student must be those that are widely generalisable and are capable of transcending a wide range of illness and wellness contexts. The professional knowledge which constitutes the specific nursing abilities of the nurse (the things that nurses do for and to the client) must be learnt in relation to solving problems for the patient and preventing problems developing.

Technical nursing skills and the problem-solving application of those skills must also be developed and nurtured from an early point in the student's training to develop the necessary attitudes and competencies that will allow her to command professional judgement and assume the appropriate accountability. The physical, behavioural and social skills that, along with the technical nursing know-how, make up the essential elements of most nursing interventions, need to be viewed for learning purposes within fairly broad conceptual perspectives. What are the preventative, restorative, adaptive and maintenance activities of nursing? These broad nursing concepts need to be seen by the student first as discrete groups of technical nursing skills and approaches that have particular value and utility within the overall care of the patient. Each element of nursing care needs to be delivered to the patient within the nursing process format of individual and personalised care. Each set of skills needs to be usable within problem-solving contexts which encourage the use of professional judgement and responsibility.

How is the patient comforted, protected, nurtured and developed by using particular nursing care concepts and their relative elements of nursing care? Within the curriculum the specific nursing knowledge must specify nursing activities which will help restore a patient's functioning to its normal level, control potential threats in the environment that would be detrimental to his health and prevent or forestall processes that would be detrimental to his health. Such knowledge and skills must also help in the adaptation of the patient to illness, return to health, or death, by adapting to the needs and problem alleviating measures with the care to be given.

The argument developing here is that the practical nursing skills of the nurse need to be viewed within quite specific parameters both for practice and educational purposes. The caring skills of the nurse, although directed at the whole patient as an individual, have independent utility and purpose and each set of skills needs to be viewed for its specific and particular purpose within any single nursing intervention.

Preventative Nursing Interventions. In preventive nursing interventions the nursing care is directed at preventing effects detrimental to the patient's health, and the nursing actions are designed to 'prevent'. In this sense they are prophylactic measures which help to check in advance the processes which lead to or precipitate health deterioration. Such activities seek to prevent ill health and so promote physical and mental health and efficiency. The nursing care elements here must identify factors which precipitate ill health or increase a person's vulnerability to ill health.

Restorative Nursing Interventions. The restorative nursing interventions are concerned with returning the patient's functioning to the normal or optimal level, that is, the best or most favourable state possible for any individual patient. This means helping the patient to renewed health or attempting to return him to a state of acceptable health. The restorative technical nursing skills include the use of techniques, methods and procedures which enable or aid the process of natural or medically aided healing. The concern of the nurse is with re-establishing or re-building patient capability whether physical, social or emotional within the activities of living.

Performing for the patient or enabling him to deal with his activities of living and providing for him while he develops the necessary strength and will to recover, depends on the ability of the nurse to identify and use appropriate methods and procedures of nursing care. The curriculum in this respect must equip the nurse with the necessary technical nursing ability to do so. The student must be able to identify and define those nursing problems which require specific restorative nursing interventions. Within the care she gives, she must be capable of assessing the significance of a whole range of factors, physical, social, personal, cultural and behavioural, which are affected when the normal health of the individual becomes disrupted by illness.

Adaptive Nursing Interventions. Adaptive nursing interventions are those nursing actions which are designed to 'adapt' the patient within certain limits with respect to his activities of living, but below full health capacity. They include the techniques and procedures that enable adaptation by the patient to his changed state during a period of ill health. They also include the adaptation of the particular environment in which the nursing care is received by the patient. The nursing events are concerned with fitting the patient to, or modifying or altering a situation, with respect to the patient's activities of living. The patient is adapted to adjust physically, socially and behaviourally to a particular situation and environment which is limiting for the patient because of his illness. The patient may have to come to terms with changes in body structure or function in a particular illness because of temporary incapacity or permanently reduced normal capacity where residual effects of illness are permanent or long-term. Considerable nursing care will be directed at attempting to adapt the patient within a certain range of disability or handicap and at the same time establish for the patient some measure of quality within his living activities. Enabling the patient to come to terms with reduced physical ability, to modify his behaviour appropriately and develop the necessary social fit or social re-adjustment, will depend on the ability of the nurse to have the correct conceptual awareness of 'adaptive' nursing actions and the necessary technical nursing skills to help the patient adjust. Such knowledge and skills must have a prominent position in the specific nursing knowledge area of the curriculum.

Maintenance Nursing Interventions. Maintenance nursing interventions are those nursing actions designed to 'maintain' the patient in an optimal state once such a state has been reached, or to prevent deterioration in the patient's general state of illness, incapacity or handicap. The emphasis of nursing activities is upon preserving the patient's condition, while supporting, sustaining and defending the patient against developing a worsened state of functional activity, disability or deterioration. The patient is maintained at a particular level of physical, social and behavioural activity until restoration to health or adaptation to limited health is achieved. The techniques and methods are those nursing actions and events which are appropriate to maintain a particular optimal level within the patient. The curriculum must accommodate realistic applications for the student of maintenance nursing activities within a problem-solving context and a nursing process format.

The Complementary Nature of Nursing Interventions. The four forms of nursing intervention described are not mutually exclusive or functionally discrete in actual practice, and they are seen in a number of established nursing models which have been reviewed in earlier chapters. The four interventions are more often than not complementary to each other and interrelated within a span of nursing care for any patient. However, there are of course appropriate situations when one particular form of nursing intervention overrides the others in terms of priority, emphasis and length of time it needs to be central to the care of the patient. There is certainly a need for the student of nursing to be able to conceptualise those nursing techniques, methods and procedures which are preventative, restorative, adaptive, or maintenance in nature and for her to be able to identify the need for specific interventions and how they can be effectively incorporated into the patient care plan. By actually identifying the specific nature of particular interventions, the nurse is able to give nursing care and use appropriate techniques with greater understanding of the reasons for the care, which will help her accountability.

The nursing curriculum, with respect to clinical nursing experience provided for the student, must prepare the student to identify and define the four types of nursing intervention and enable the student to use the general concepts of each intervention in her learning experience in the clinical settings. The use of the four types of nursing intervention must also be taught in such a way that the student becomes a member of the ward team and sees her involvement in the care of patients as part of an overall health team approach to patient care. As other members of the health care team, including medical and paramedical groups, are equally concerned with notions of 'prevention', 'restoring', 'adapting' and 'maintaining', there is a need for the student to learn and experience the interdependency factor which is necessary to give the patient all of the available health care expertise he requires. Nursing care is a particular form of caring expertise, but it is not exclusive, nor is the care of the patient exclusively the domain of any particular health worker over and above the involvement of others. The curriculum, in the way it deals with the specific nursing knowledge and skills, must take account of the way in which such knowledge and skills relates to other health care occupational groups both in terms of the differences and the similarities.

Nursing Process

In addition to the antecedent knowledge of nursing and the specific nursing knowledge, the nursing process can be used as an organising theme by drawing on the antecedent subjects basic to nursing, and by giving ordered and rational applications of nursing interventions and events within the nursing curriculum.

The most useful approach is to use the nursing process at three levels of increasing difficulty from its simplest form of standard care plan and basic nursing approaches to its most sophisticated and complex form. Three levels of application would also logically be applied to the three years of nurse education required for State Registration. This chronological use of the process may be outlined as follows:

(i) 1st Level – 1st Year of Training. Emphasis on the nursing process at a basic level and its application to individual patients using standard care plans and personalised adaptations to individual patients in a varied and comprehensive series of nursing contexts.

(ii) 2nd Level – 2nd Year of Training. Emphasis at this level is on the application of the nursing process using greater complexities of technical, behavioural and social skills. The applications of the nursing process are studied in depth and heavier demands are made on the student's cognitive, affective and psycho-motor abilities, to develop skills in prediction, analysis and evaluation as modes of more sophisticated problem-solving.

(iii) 3rd Level – 3rd Year of Training. Emphasis is on sophisticated use and application of the nursing process. Broader dimensions can be added in such a way as to develop leadership and professional responsibility in the student. Theoretical frames of reference can be used from several nursing models to formulate nursing care plans and interventions. Analysis of individual patient nursing contexts is therefore made from several theoretical positions and applications made to broad specialisms to individuals and groups of patients.

The Nursing Process as an Educational Tool within the Curriculum. In the hands of experienced teachers and using the nursing process as a broad conceptual framework for the curriculum, it is possible to develop both intellectual and practical skills in the learner nurse and, at the same time, develop scientific approaches to the care of patients. The underlying purpose here would be the development of a nurse that can incorporate into her nursing repertoire the ability to seek and solve problems.

The student of nursing should be able to participate in the individual nursing care of a patient and, at the same time, make a fairly in-depth study of the individualised care she gives. The logical format involved would be problem-solving based on scientific method and the emphasis would be on observing, recording, analysing and evaluating nursing care as well as simply effecting the delivery of that care. In such contexts the nursing process can be looked upon and used as an educational tool as well as an organisational means towards individual patient care, and the process in effect can be viewed by the teacher and the curriculum organiser as a major frame of reference for learning purposes.

Using the nursing process as a problem-solving approach can also take into account the student's developing theoretical knowledge of biological and behavioural science and their practical application to nursing care. Observations and inferences made by the student should be focused on biological and behavioural responses of the patient to stress, therapeutic effect, nursing actions and events. Much data will emerge from student/patient interactions which need to be accurately recorded, carefully analysed and systematically ordered by the student. A written record with reasoned and justified accounts of the care given could be developed in respect of individual patients, and this would form a continuous learning experience of giving care to patients and a meaningful record of that care. In this way, the student acts as a participant and observer in patient care. Careful monitoring by the teacher of the student/patient interaction would be needed and both teacher and student would collaborate on analysis of the data and the effects of the patient care.

The objectives of such problem-solving events within patient care would allow the student to make in-depth and continuous analysis of her nursing care experiences and provide her with a permanent record of problem-solving action in the clinical area in which she is currently gaining experience.

Such learning events would allow the development of logical answers or generalisations by explaining relationships based on facts obtained through observation (inductive reasoning). The student could also gain practice in developing logical answers or conclusions from reliable premises using general propositions to derive the right conclusions (deductive reasoning). In both instances the provision of evidence of the extent to which the student understands the clinical nursing events analysed would be available for the teacher.

Within such learning contexts, certain principles would be applied to the overall learning experience of the student.

First the student identifies, collects and analyses data related to a series of nursing care problems presented by the patient. Secondly, the student determines scientific reasons for these problems. Thirdly, she makes descriptions, analyses and hypotheses of the nursing care given, with supporting data. Fourthly, she attempts to determine scientific reasons for the nursing care she has given.

In the inductive approach, principles are developed after consideration of the facts of individual patient problems. In the deductive approach the reverse applies and the principles serve as means of interpreting facts. In practice, induction and deduction are inseparable, except in the simplest of problems. Professional nurses should be able to recognise and apply both inductive and deductive procedures in the solution of certain types of problems, and in the planning and adopting of procedures to be followed. Irrespective of whether the problem is essentially of the deductive or the inductive type, the practical procedure is much the same. The real difference is not in the method of procedure but in the nature of the outcomes of the thinking.

It is essential in the overall scheme of the curriculum to view the nursing process theme, not simply as an integrating mechanism for relating theoretical assumptions about nursing and nursing practice itself, but as a way of developing in the student particular modes of thinking and a capability to be creative in dealing with patients' problems.

The Educational Application of the Nursing Process to Clinical Work Experience for the Student of Nursing. Within the operational curriculum the student of nursing should, in the clinical settings she is allocated to for experience in nursing patients, be able to function as both a participant in patient care and an observer of patient care. The student should also at the same time be able to make objective and scientific analyses of the nursing care she is involved in and produce a data record for her own study purposes. The essential and predominant feature of the record would be to secure a critical systematic analysis of the nursing care and its effects upon the patients by using a scientific method of approach in an attempt to understand the nature of the care. In this sense the student will be a participant in the care of patients and will make an in-depth study of individual nursing care and the processes applied to effect that care.

The main approach would be one of problem-solving directly related to individualised approaches to nursing care which are characterised through the use of the nursing process. The nursing process would be the theoretical frame of reference for the student and the practical frame of operation for the nursing care involved. The investigatory approach by the student would be by objective data gathering, analysis and evaluation with an ultimate attempt to synthesise data about activities of nursing care. The student would require teacher supervision by a nurse educator who has retained the clinical skills of a practising nurse or by a practising clinical nurse who has acquired the skills of teaching in the clinical setting. The student would be involved in the supervised care of the patient and would be given sufficient time over the working day to make the necessary observations and collections of data.

In this respect the student would be expected to observe, analyse, record, synthesise and evaluate activities of nursing care and their effects upon the patient and his problems.

These observations and analytic activities would take into account the student's developing theoretical knowledge of biology, behavioural science, pathology, technical nursing skills and their practical application to individualised nursing care. The observations made by the student would particularly consider the biological and behavioural responses of the patients to nursing events and actions. The data collected by the student from observations made during nursing events would be accurately recorded, systematically analysed and provide objective study data for the student's own written clinical nursing record. A meaningful nursing record and a reasoned and justified account of the student's interpretation of the care she has been involved in would emerge to form the basis for student-teacher discussion and evaluation.

The following general objectives would be useful guidelines for both students and teachers in applying such a problem-solving framework as an educational tool, and at the same time allowing experience to be gained in using the nursing process:

Objectives

(1) To allow students to make an in-depth and continuous analysis of their nursing care experiences in the clinical nursing setting.
(2) To provide for the student an objective account and record of problem-solving experiences related to the nursing care given to patients during allocations to clinical experience areas.
(3) To give the student practice in developing logical answers or generalisations by explaining relationships based on facts obtained through participant observation (inductive approach).
(4) To give the student practice in developing logical answers or conclusions from reliable premises using general propositions to derive conclusions obtained through participant observation (deductive approach).
(5) To provide evidence of the extent to which the student understands the clinical nursing events analysed.

The student should have a known problem-solving approach that will help to formulate a procedure for tackling problems. This usually involves identifying a problem, defining it and delimiting it to realistic and manageable proportions. Several possible solutions might be proposed (the statement of hypotheses), but only one hypothesis is selected at any one time for testing. The student makes a systematic attempt to collect and organise relevant information and uses the logical processes of induction, deduction and judgement (makes a critical evaluation) according to their relevance to the problem and the data. The student then attempts to arrive at a solution which is appropriate and reasonable by logical processes and then attempts to verify the solution and justify the conclusions.

This fairly standard scientific approach requires student-teacher collaboration to develop proficiency in the student in the problem-solving events. Attention needs to be focused on reducing initial problems to writing and stating problems clearly and precisely. The statements need to be in quite specific terms which allow for only one possible meaning or interpretation, rather than using general words or nursing jargon. The meaning of all words must be meaningful and free from possible misinterpretation. Careful limitation of general problems needs to be done and irrelevant material discarded. Complex problems must be reduced by dividing them into several separate discrete problems. Where problems are not clear, students need to discuss these carefully with the teacher and additional reading may then be necessary before approaching the problems again. The student may then propose a solution or sets of solutions by setting up hypotheses. The teacher, in collaboration with the student, needs to guide the student in gathering data and organising the data as well as assisting the student in proving solutions to the problems and in checking and verifying solutions.

Nursing Process – Problem-solving Activities. Some Guidelines

The compilation of data, descriptions and analyses made by the student for her study record should appropriately take account of a nursing process approach as the problem-solving format in the approach to the study of nursing care. The four major recognised stages of the nursing process, (1) assessment, (2) planning, (3) implementation and (4) evaluation, should be taken as the four essential perspectives of nursing care in which problems should be located and dealt with by systematic investigation. To this end the nursing process should be considered as the focal frame of reference, and problems arising within it should be viewed from a biological, behavioural and pathological set of inferences (as well as technical nursing) supported by the currently emerging nursing concepts taken from appropriate nursing models. The overall point of the exercise would be to make theoretically informed inferences about the problems of patients and the way in which individualised nursing care was identified, used and reasoned to be appropriate for the patient and effective in reducing his problems.

Assessment. For the assessment phase of the nursing process, emphasis should be placed on developing the theoretical and practical ability of the student to assess the patient's physical, behavioural and social needs. This involves the student in attempting to make a comprehensive theoretical and actual patient assessment by defining and identifying the patient's range of physical, emotional and social problems by developing a data base and using known data bases. The student would select and use appropriate data gathering guides and methods and determine the correct way to analyse and synthesise the data. Identification of an individual patient's needs and problems by determining actual and potential problems would be necessary, as would correctly discriminating between usual and unusual problems and needs. The student might make statements about the cause and effects of the patient's condition and make concise notes on any appropriate and relevant scientific facts in relationship to each problem identified. By interviewing the patient and obtaining a nursing history, necessary data would be obtained from which the student could specify, define and clarify the patient's problems logically. The student might also describe and justify the nature of the interview and other data collecting approaches she uses, and describe the mode and nature of the communication processes used and the patient's responses.

Planning. For the planning phase of the nursing process, emphasis should be placed on developing the theoretical and practical ability of the student to make theoretically supported practical applications in planning nursing care strategies. Following the previous systematic review of patient data, definition and classification of problems, the nature and form of care to be given is broadly determined and nursing care priorities established. Nursing care objectives in the short, medium and long term are decided and the objective statements made, justified by a reasoned analysis. The student needs to consider the possible choices available and then come to an appropriate decision which is correct for a particular problem. Determining appropriate measuring criteria for the nursing care objectives would help determine the validity of approach to the planning phase. The student can now arrive at a basic framework of a plan for the patient which can be viewed as the 'standard care plan' initially. Following consultation with other nurses involved in the patient's care, and other team members (including the medical staff involved) and the patient himself, an individualised nursing care plan is produced. The plan is shaped by determining the scope and sequence of nursing events, and justified by giving a reasoned account of scope and sequence, the ranking and ordering of nursing care needs and actions. At this point it is necessary to give some thought to determining the process to measure the quality of the intended nursing care based on some valid criteria.

Implementation. For the implementation phase of the nursing process, emphasis should be placed upon developing the student's ability to make theoretically supported practical applications in implementing nursing care strategies. For study and learning purposes the student should be able to describe how she has managed and co-ordinated the planned nursing events and describe and justify the nature of communication used with the patient and other care givers during the implementation of the nursing care. Descriptions and analyses by the student about how she has used and controlled appropriate resources used in the care of the patient would be desirable along with explanations concerning her approaches in monitoring and maintaining care. It would be useful also for the student to identify and describe changes in the implementation of care that were different from the original planned nursing activities, and for her to account for the reasons and need to make changes. Within the continuous delivery of care during the implementation phase, identification of critical incidents and a critical reasoned account of the nursing measures taken to alleviate the problems are singularly important items for the student's written record. Within the delivery of nursing to the patient the use of particular nursing skills and technology is important in terms of justifying their use and effect along with a careful analysis of the nature of nursing events, whether restorative, maintenance, adaptive or rehabilitative. Finally, consideration of the patient's behavioural, physical and emotional responses to nursing care will provide a wealth of observable and recordable data from which important inferences and conclusions may be reached.

Evaluation. For the evaluation phase of the nursing process, emphasis should be placed upon developing the student's ability to evaluate the effectiveness of the nursing care that has been planned and implemented. This means involving the student in the making of both qualitative and quantifiable evaluations of nursing care and the making of decisions to alter care on the basis of appropriate and relevant findings. The student will need to select and use appropriate evaluation procedures to observe the intended and unintended results of nursing care. This will involve the student in the development of skills necessary to perceive, observe and analyse the planned nursing events and the critical incidents occurring. She will need to know and make use of data feedback mechanisms which will demonstrate effected changes to the form, nature and quality of care. Ability to be able to differentiate between qualitative and quantifiable approaches and objectivity in the evaluation of nursing care will be a significant gain in learning for the student. Primarily, making use of selective specified procedures of evaluation and differentiating between formative and summative approaches would be necessary skills for the student in evaluating complex nursing care events, over both the long and short term. The ability to record evaluated findings accurately and act on information gained to make decisions related to the outcomes of nursing care will also be desirable skills for the student to develop. The student should master a wide and comprehensive range of data collecting, analysis and synthesis procedures, suitable for subjective and objective aspects of nursing care evaluation. The observation of intended and unintended results of the use of the nursing process as a whole through the use of evaluatory rating scales, check lists, systematic observation, verbal and written reports of involved staff, should be considered essential formats for analysis, and important sources from which to make evaluatory judgements and assist in achieving quality standards of nursing care.

The methods so far outlined for using the nursing process as a specific educational tool in developing in students a scientific approach to thinking about nursing care, are used at the author's own college, Liverpool Polytechnic, for students taking the Diploma in Professional Studies in Nursing. There is no logical reason why similar methods cannot be used in schools of nursing at the pre-registration level in the preparation of nurses for clinical nursing practice.

(iii) The Curriculum Matrix

The curriculum matrix in this book is used as an instrument to help in the planning of the curriculum and decision-making about objectives, content, methods and evaluation aspects of the nursing curriculum in respect of the nursing process.The matrix is represented by sixteen frames which attempt to interrelate the four phases of the curriculum process in a vertical dimension and the four phases of the nursing process in a horizontal dimension. In this way the assessment, planning, implementation and evaluation phases are shown in horizontal alignment and the objectives, content, methods and evaluation phases of the curriculum process are shown in vertical alignment.

Each individual frame represents a potential area of identification of elements of the nursing process and the curriculum process by which decisions can be made regarding the curriculum arrangements. For example, frame 1.2 relates to the curriculum objectives for the planning phase of the nursing process. Similarly, frame 3.3 relates to the curriculum methods to be used for the implementation phase of the nursing process, and frame 4.1 relates to the curriculum evaluation of the assessment phase of the nursing process, and so on (see Table 1).

The matrix could easily be adapted for use in the determination of scope, sequence and integration of content, but that is not the intention in this particular study. The intention here is to show a total relationship of the curriculum process to the nursing process for curricular planning decision-making reasons.

The total relationship of curriculum process and nursing process is shown in Table 1, and Table 2 shows the specific cross-relationships of the phases of the nursing process to the phases of the curriculum process represented within the nursing curriculum matrix.

The matrix does not do anything of itself, but it does allow the curriculum designer and planner to focus thinking in two dimensions on particular areas of the curriculum. The two dimensions concerned here are the phases of the curriculum process and the phases of the nursing process. These can be brought together to pinpoint areas of concern in the curriculum.

The following worked example may help to illustrate how the matrix can be used.

Suppose for example the planner was concerned with curriculum content (that is, particular subject material) and the particular content in question was part of the syllabus dealing with 'pain' and how the nurse deals with this in the assessment phase of the nursing process. Pain would be located as content on the matrix and its relationship would be in line with the assessment, 2.1, as shown in Table 1. The following deductions could be made for instance on the perception of pain.

Example: 'The Perception of Pain'

Assessment

(1) Assessment of type, location and quality of pain.
(2) Assessment of intensity of pain, nature of onset and precipitating factors.
(3) Assessing aggravating factors, associated factors and alleviating factors.

Table 1: The Nursing Curriculum Matrix, Showing the Total Relationship of the Curriculum Process and the Nursing Process

VERTICAL DIMENSION CURRICULUM PROCESS	HORIZONTAL DIMENSION NURSING PROCESS				
	NURSING CURRICULUM MATRIX	PHASE ONE ASSESSMENT	PHASE TWO PLANNING	PHASE THREE IMPLEMENTATION	PHASE FOUR EVALUATION
	PHASE ONE OBJECTIVES	1.1	1.2	1.3	1.4
	PHASE TWO CONTENT	2.1	2.2	2.3	2.4
	PHASE THREE METHODS	3.1	3.2	3.3	3.4
	PHASE FOUR EVALUATION	4.1	4.2	4.3	4.4

Table 2: The Interrelationship of the Curriculum Process and the Nursing Process within the Nursing Curriculum Matrix

CURRICULUM	NURSING PROCESS
CURRICULUM OBJECTIVES	
PHASE 1.1	The learning objectives required in the *assessment phase* of the nursing process
PHASE 1.2	The learning objectives required in the *planning phase* of the nursing process
PHASE 1.3	The learning objectives required in the *implementation phase* of the nursing process
PHASE 1.4	The learning objectives required in the *evaluation phase* of the nursing process
CURRICULUM CONTENT	
PHASE 2.1	The identification and selection of curricular content for the *assessment phase* of the nursing process
PHASE 2.2	The identification and selection of curricular content for the *planning phase* of the nursing process
PHASE 2.3	The identification and selection of curricular content for the *implementation phase* of the nursing process
PHASE 2.4	The identification and selection of curricular content for the *evaluation phase* of the nursing process
CURRICULUM METHODS	
PHASE 3.1	The instructional methods to be used and learning experiences to be created for the *assessment phase* of the nursing process
PHASE 3.2	The instructional methods to be used and learning experiences to be created for the *planning phase* of the nursing process
PHASE 3.3	The instructional methods to be used and learning experiences to be created for the *implementation phase* of the nursing process
PHASE 3.4	The instructional methods to be used and learning experiences to be created for the *evaluation phase* of the nursing process
CURRICULUM EVALUATION	
PHASE 4.1	The curriculum evaluation of the *assessment phase* of the nursing process
PHASE 4.2	The curriculum evaluation of the *planning phase* of the nursing process
PHASE 4.3	The curriculum evaluation of the *implementation phase* of the nursing process
PHASE 4.4	The curriculum evaluation of the *evaluation phase* of the nursing process

(4) Assessing patients' behavioural responses to pain.

In this example part of the curriculum content, 'the perception of pain', has been related to the assessment factors which would be used in caring for the patient using the nursing process approach. The matrix has allowed identification of the relevant assessment procedures in relationship to the perception of pain.

A further example might be where the planner is still concentrating on 'the perception of pain' as the relevant content area of the curriculum, but now deals with pain in the implementation phase of the nursing process. In this situation pain is again located as content on the matrix but its relationship would be in line with the implementation, 2.3, as shown in Table 1. The following deductions could be made for instance on the perception of pain from an implementation perspective.

Example: 'The Perception of Pain'

Implementation

(1) Provision of nursing interventions that provide pain relief.
(2) Alleviating pain through touch.
(3) Alleviating pain through the use of heat and cold.
(4) Achieving pain relief using medications.
(5) Teaching the patient methods to reduce pain.
(6) Achieving pain relief using relaxation methods.
(7) Considering research studies of pain relief.

In this example part of the curriculum content, 'the perception of pain', has been related to the nursing interventions which would be appropriate in the implementation phase of the nursing process in dealing with a patient's pain.

Still concentrating on 'pain' as the example of part of the curriculum, the matrix could now be used to identify curriculum objectives and these objectives could be set in relationship to the assessment phase of the nursing process. In this instance the focus of the matrix would be on 1.1, as shown in Table 1.

Example: 'The Perception of Pain'

Learning Objectives for Assessment of Patients with Pain

(1) The student will be able to identify the type, location and quality of pain.

(2) The student will be able to identify the degree of intensity of pain, nature of onset, length of duration, and determine precipitating factors.
(3) The student will be able to identify specific aggravating factors, factors associated with the pain, and factors tending to alleviate or reduce the pain.
(4) The student will be able to identify changes in the patient's behaviour that are directly related to the nature of the pain.

In this instance appropriate learning objectives have been identified by which the student can concentrate on developing assessment skills related to her perception of the patient's pain within the assessment phase of the nursing process.

(iv) The Relationship of the Curriculum Process to the Nursing Process

The broad conceptual relationships are shown in Table 2, in which curriculum objectives, content, methods and evaluation are shown schematically in relationship or alignment to the nursing process. The intention is to demonstrate the need for each phase of the nursing process to be looked at in terms of preparing suitable curriculum objectives, curricular content (subject matter to be taught and learnt), curricular methods (how the teaching and learning is to be organised) and curricular evaluation (how the teaching and learning is evaluated).

For instance, phase 1.1, in Table 2, shows that for the assessment phase of the nursing process certain curriculum objectives need to be decided for the direction of the student learning. Phases 1.2, 1.3 and 1.4 are similarly related to planning, implementation and evaluation of nursing care.

In phases 2.1 to 2.4, the focus is on deciding which content (subject matter) should be selected and included in the curriculum and how a detailed expansion of material might be done, again in relationship to the four elements of the nursing process.

In phase 3.1 to 3.4, the focus is on selecting, preparing and using appropriate teaching and learning materials and approaches, that would be suitable for dealing with subject matter concerned with nursing process approaches to the care of patients.

In phases 4.1 to 4.4, the focus is on attempting to decide how the teaching and learning of the nursing process approach to nursing care can be evaluated, and which evaluation arrangements and procedures are most appropriate.

An overview is now presented on curriculum objectives and how they relate to the nursing process, curriculum content, methods and evaluation, and how they each relate to the nursing process. Each of these is also represented in tables to show some of the specific curriculum activities in relationship to aspects of nursing care within the nursing process. Activities, assignments and intended instructional events are presented as guidelines for curricular decision making.

(v) Curriculum Objectives and the Nursing Process

The relationship of the curriculum objectives represented as phase one is shown in alignment to the four elements of the nursing process in Figure 4. In the assessment of individual patients for nursing care interventions, identification of needs and the diagnosing of actual and potential problems will be required on clear statements of learning objectives. Learning objectives will also be required to develop the perception and observational skills in the student in order to make accurate and informed observations of patients. As interviewing and communicating with patients are central features of assessment and diagnostic statements of learning, objectives will also be required for these. Objectives will also need to be designed to develop the student's abilities to discriminate and analyse complex data about the patient ranging from behavioural to social and physical aspects.

In the planning of individual patient care, statements of learning objectives will be required to develop the student's ability to identify possible solutions to patients' problems and, in doing so, analyse the situation for nursing options and make decisions regarding the choice of options. The central element of the planning phase concerns the formulation of nursing care plans and the development of criteria for nursing events within the plans. Learning objectives will be required to develop planning skills in the student's repertoire of abilities and will include effective communication of the intentions of the plan to all nursing staff involved in the care of the patient.

In the implementation of individual patient care, learning objectives will need to be prepared to enable the student to institute specific nursing skills and techniques in accordance with the plan of care. Personalised approaches and the maintenance of effective rapport and communication will be important aspects for learning objectives. Objectives will also be needed to develop abilities in the student to control the nursing events and develop overall co-ordination of the total patient care. Monitoring nursing events and modifying nursing objectives through effective feedback mechanisms will also require clear learning objectives for the student. Within the implementation phase, students will learn how to teach patients self-care, and objectives will be needed to prepare students for this teaching role.

Figure 4: Phase One: The Relationship of Curriculum Objectives to the Four Elements of the Nursing Process.

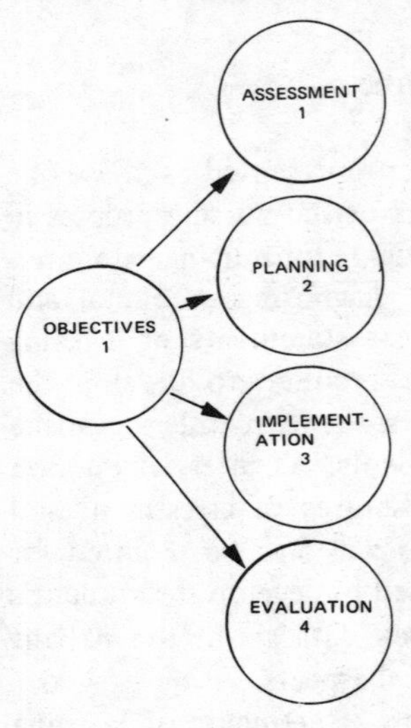

The evaluation of individual nursing care will require the student to be able to make formative and summative assessments of nursing care and recognise and use both objective and subjective aspects of evaluation. Learning objectives will need to be developed so that the student can decide on the recording and communication strategies required in evaluating nursing care. This must also include analysing and synthesising data, developing awareness and ability to make necessary changes in nursing events, and setting new nursing objectives in the light of evaluation outcomes. There must also be learning objectives to enable the student to identify critical incidents in nursing events that have bearing and influence on the quality of nursing care. The curriculum objectives are essential prerequisites in curriculum planning regarding the form and intentions of the curriculum as a whole and its relationship to the nursing process. Table 3 gives examples of aspects of the nursing process for which learning objectives will be required.

Table 3: Curriculum Objectives and the Nursing Process

Assessment

Statements of objectives for:

(i) identifying patient needs.
(ii) identifying and diagnosing patient problems, actual and potential.
(iii) perception and observation of the patient.
(iv) interviewing and communication with the patient.
(v) discrimination and analysis of data about the patient.

Planning

Statements of objectives for:

(i) identification of possible solutions to patient problems.
(ii) analysing nursing options.
(iii) deciding choice of options.
(iv) formulation of the nursing care plan and deciding criteria.
(v) communication of the purposes of the plan to all staff.

Implementation

Statements of objectives for:

(i) instituting specific nursing skill and techniques.
(ii) maintaining a personalised approach.
(iii) developing and maintaining effective rapport and communication.
(iv) focusing care toward potential and expected outcomes.
(v) co-ordination of the nursing events to control interventions.
(vi) monitoring the nursing events and modifying objectives of care.
(vii) providing feedback of nursing care outcomes to the patient and the nursing team.
(viii) teaching the patient self-care.

Evaluation

Statements of objectives for:

(i) making formative and summative assessments of nursing care.
(ii) identifying methods (objective and subjective) for the assessment of nursing events and patient responses to nursing care.
(iii) deciding the recording and communication strategies.
(iv) analysing and synthesising data.
(v) identifying the need to make changes in the nursing care.
(vi) setting new nursing objectives in the light of evaluation outcomes.
(vii) identifying critical incidents in the nursing events with respect to the quality of nursing care.

(vi) Curriculum Content and the Nursing Process

The relationship of the curriculum content stage of the curriculum process represented as phase two is shown in alignment to the four elements of the nursing process in Figure 5. In the assessment phase of the nursing process, students must have access to knowledge and develop understanding of processes and sources of data collection and identify relevance and validity of specific data with respect to individual patients. Similarly the student must be able to analyse, sequence and synthesise patient data which have been obtained as evidence of an individual patient's needs and problems in a wide range of nursing contexts. Data which the nurse collects must be efficiently and clearly documented for communication and record purposes.

The techniques of interviewing and history-taking are central to the assessment phase for nursing diagnosis and must include perceptual and observational skills related to the physical, behavioural and social considerations of the patient.

Figure 5: Phase Two: The Relationship of Curriculum Content to the Four Elements of the Nursing Process.

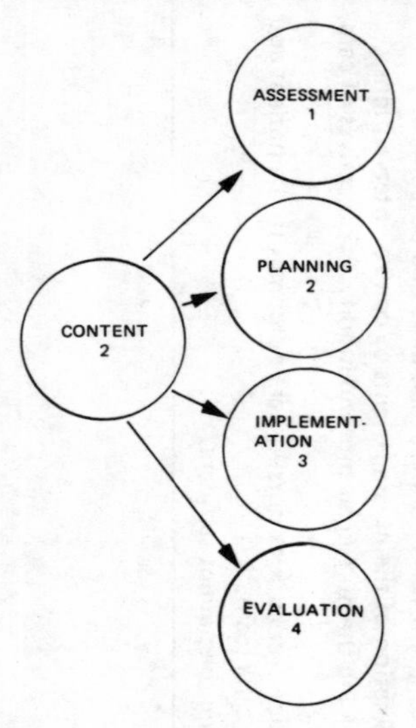

The content of the curriculum should also include the appropriate strategic aspects of nursing care planning that allow reinforcement of individualised and personalised aspects of nursing care and as such take account of similarities and differences between individual patients in respect of their unique health problems. The planning of care must also clearly be seen in terms of its problem-solving context, and students must be able to apply problem-solving skills to the production of basic (standard) nursing care plans and specific individualised care plans in varied and diverse nursing situations.

The content of the curriculum in relationship to the implementation of the nursing process should be concerned with the specific nursing technologies and skills used in nursing interventions and must include decision-making related to choices available about the kinds of care to be implemented. Control of the immediate environment of patients, effective use of available resources, and the management, control and co-ordination of individual patient care events will be central areas of concern. A major emphasis will also need to be made on teaching patients self-care.

The content of the curriculum with respect to patient care evaluation must deal with conceptualisations of evaluation and assessment and make clear the necessary distinctions between these. Values and standards and qualitative and quantifiable aspects of evaluating will also need to be dealt with, as will the necessary distinction between objective and subjective approaches. Formative and summative forms of evaluation and the identification, selection and use of evaluation procedures will be central features of the content of the curriculum. The overriding fundamental requirement for the evaluation phase of the nursing process must be seen as the ability of the nurse to make effective judgements about the safety, quality and standard of care and, where necessary, effect changes in the light of feedback during the monitoring of the nursing events. Table 4 gives examples of curriculum content in respect of the four phases of the nursing process and they are not offered as being mutually exclusive or exhaustive.

(vii) Curriculum Methods and the Nursing Process

The relationship of the curriculum method stage of the curriculum process represented as phase three is shown in alignment to the four elements of the nursing process in Figure 6. The emphasis on method throughout the nursing curriculum in respect of the nursing process should be concerned with active learning events and the operationalisation of learning objectives and content areas by intended instructional events and learning experiences for the students. For the assessment

Table 4: Curriculum Content and the Nursing Process

Assessment	Planning
Identification of content to develop the technical, behavioural and intellectual skills required in the assessment of patients in diversified nursing care settings.	Identification of content to develop the technical, behavioural and intellectual skills required to plan nursing care in varied and diversified nursing care settings.
(i) The process of data collection.	(i) Learning care planning skills using concepts of individualised and personalised care.
(ii) Awareness of data sources.	(ii) Taking account of similarities and differences in patients with respect to needs and problems of a social, emotional and physical form.
(iii) Relevance and validity of data.	(iii) Standard care plans (basic plans) and the elements of nursing care that are likely to be applicable to most patients.
(iv) Analysis, sequencing and the synthesis of data.	(iv) Problem-solving sequences in the development of nursing care plans.
(v) Obtaining evidence of problems.	(v) Deciding specific nursing actions or nursing events and the production of a written nursing strategy.
(vi) Making needs assessments of patients, in various contexts.	(vi) Developing criteria for standards of care in standard (basic) care plans.
(vii) Documenting data base information.	
(viii) Interviewing the patient and history taking.	
(ix) Making nursing diagnoses.	
(x) Observation and perception of the patient's physical, emotional and social problems, in varying clinical contexts.	

Table 4 (continued)

Implementation

Planning put to action. Nursing interventions and nursing events that focus on the needs and problems of the individual patient. Developing in the student the technical, behavioural and intellectual skills required to implement and control planned nursing events.

(i) Making decisions about nursing events in varying and diverse nursing contexts.

(ii) Recognising and taking account of the environment of the patient.

(iii) Motivating patients and developing effective rapport and communication.

(iv) Managing and co-ordinating the planned nursing events in varied nursing contexts.

(v) Teaching patients self-care.

(vi) Meeting physical, emotional and social needs of patients.

(vii) Determining and using the correct nursing skills and techniques in the nursing interactions.

Evaluation

Identification and selection of content to develop the technical, behavioural and intellectual skills required to evaluate the nursing care of patients.

(i) The concepts of evaluation and assessment.

(ii) Values and standards in evaluation.

(iii) Qualitative and quantifiable aspects of evaluation.

(iv) Objective and subjective evaluation of nursing care.

(v) Formative and summative evaluation in nursing care.

(vi) Various methods used in the assessment of patient care.

(vii) Methods of recording data.

(viii) Methods of analysing and synthesising nursing data.

(ix) Acting on information and decision-making related to the outcomes of evaluation.

(x) Analysis of critical incidents in nursing care.

(xi) Effecting changes in nursing care in the light of feedback during the monitoring of nursing events.

phase of the nursing process, emphasis should be placed on developing student abilities to assess the patient's physical, behavioural and social problems in the widest possible range of nursing contexts. For the planning phase of the nursing process, emphasis should be placed on developing student abilities to make theoretically supported practical applications in planning nursing care strategies. For the implementation phase of the nursing process, emphasis should be placed on developing student abilities to use and operationalise the nursing care plans into actual individual nursing interventions in the widest possible range of nursing contexts. For the evaluation phase of the nursing process, emphasis should be placed on developing student abilities in evaluating the effectiveness of the care that has been planned and implemented.

Figure 6: Phase Three: The Relationship of Curricular Methods to the Four Elements of the Nursing Process.

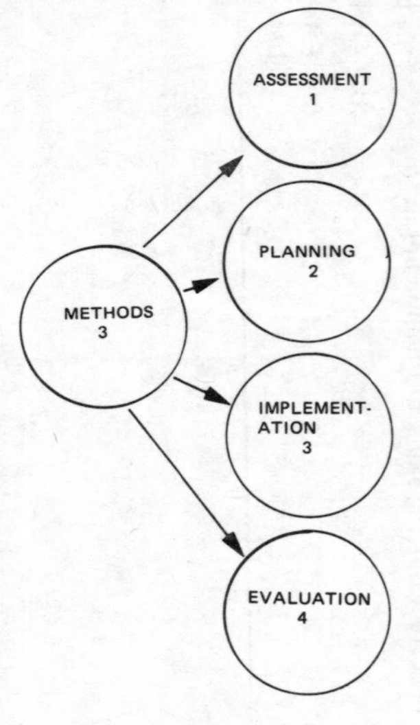

It is the author's considered opinion that the intended instructional events and learning experiences should reflect a high proportion of small-group collaborative learning activities and individualised independent learning approaches, though not exclusively so. Framework programmes of lectures would be needed for introducing areas of work and dealing with generalisations, major principles and theoretical positions related to each area of the nursing process. Small-group activities, paired student assignments and individual assignments supported by a high level of teacher involvement in the sense of facilitating and guiding functions would be a dominant format of method. Thus, tutorials with individual students and small groups, discussion groups, seminars, simulation exercises, role-play activity and collaborative workshop activities using problem-solving approaches would be appropriate methods. Nursing conferences, individual patient care studies, nursing teaching rounds, on-going instruction and supervision of students in real clinical settings will be essential components of the curriculum. In essence a high level of teacher support in patient-centred situations using instruction, demonstration, role modelling and supervised student practice in wards and departments is essential to the overall introduction of the nursing process approach to patient care.

The proportion of classroom teaching should not be greater than the amount of directly supervised clinical work and the clinical work must be directed toward actual patient care. Classroom work and independent learning will also need to be supported by current and appropriate educational technology with particular emphasis on information processing and problem-solving activity.

Table 5 gives examples of instructional events and learning activities appropriate for the nursing process, but is not necessarily an exhaustive list or exclusive.

Table 5: Curriculum Methods and the Nursing Process

Assessment

The identification and selection of instructional events and the creation of learning experiences to develop the technical, behavioural and intellectual skills required in the assessment of patients in diversified nursing care settings.

Intended Instructional Events

Major Focus — Problem-solving activities and information processing.

(i) Tutorials — individual and group.
(ii) Tutor-led discussion groups.
(iii) Student-led discussion groups.
(iv) Collaborative workshop group activities on selected problems.
(v) Simulation exercises using role play in selected nursing care contexts.
(vi) Assignment to selected patients in real clinical settings.
(vii) Nursing care planning conferences focussed on assessment of patients.

Intended Learning Experiences

Focus — Making comprehensive theoretical and actual patient assessments. Defining a complete range of physical, emotional and social problems for a varied range of assigned patients.

(i) Retrieving data from known data sources.
(ii) Making and selecting effective data gathering guides and demonstrating how data are secured by interview, inspection and observation of patients.
(iii) Taking nursing histories and in various patient care contexts.

continued

Table 5 (continued)

Intended Instructional Events	Intended Learning Experiences
(viii) Seminars using student prepared papers on topics of patient assessment and nursing diagnosis.	(iv) Determining and using correct procedures in analysis, sequence and synthesis of patient data. (v) Determining the nature of patient problems and making individual needs assessments to arrive at a nursing diagnosis. (vi) Correctly discriminating between usual and unusual situations for a selected number of descriptive patient care situations. (vii) Making statements of cause and effect of each problem identified and considering scientific facts related to the problems including the cause.

Planning

The identification, creation and selection of instructional events and learning experiences to develop the technical, behavioural and intellectual skills required to plan nursing care in varied and diverse nursing care settings.

Intended Instructional Events	Intended Learning Experiences
Major Focus — Information processing and problem solving. (i) Tutorials, individual and group. (ii) Tutor-led discussion groups. (iii) Student-led discussion groups. (iv) Collaborative workshop group activities on selected planning aspects of nursing care. (v) Nursing care conferences, multi-disciplinary approaches with the presence of selected patients and patient data. (vi) Simulation exercises using role play in planning nursing care in selected nursing care contexts. (vii) Assignment of students to selected patients in real clinical settings, with focus on nursing care planning. (viii) Seminars using student prepared papers on topics of nursing care planning. (ix) Role-play exercises in the communication aspects of nursing care planning.	*Focus* — Making comprehensive theoretical and actual patient care plans to develop nursing care|planning skills. (i) Reviewing and examining data systematically. Specifying, defining and classifying problems logically. (ii) Determining scope and sequence in nursing events. Ranking and ordering nursing care needs. Identifying priorities. (iii) Setting nursing care intentions and purposes by determining short, medium and long term objectives of nursing care. (iv) Using decision-making skills in the formulation of nursing care plans. (v) Setting criteria for measuring the achievement of nursing care intentions. (vi) Production of written standard (basic) nursing care plans.

continued

Table 5 (continued)

Intended Learning Experiences

(vii) Production of written individual (unique) nursing care plans.
(viii) Consultation and collaboration with care team members in the negotiation of individual care plans.
(ix) Communication (written and oral) to explain intentions of individual nursing care plans.
(x) Plan.

Implementation

The identification, creation and selection of instructional events and learning experiences to develop the technical, behavioural and intellectual skills required to implement individual nursing care events in varied and diverse nursing care settings.

Intended Instructional Events

Major Focus — Application to the delivery of nursing care — the elements of problem solving

(i) Simulation exercises using role play in selected and varied nursing care contexts.
(ii) Assignment to selected patients in real clinical settings.
(iii) Tutorials, individual and group.
(iv) Tutor-led discussion groups.
(v) Student-led discussion groups.
(vi) Seminars using students' prepared papers on topics of nursing care delivery.
(vii) Collaborative work-group activities on selected aspects of nursing care implementation for specific individual patients.
(viii) Nursing care conferences using multi-disciplinary approaches with the presence of selected patients and/or patient data related to the delivery of nursing care.
(ix) Role-play (modelling) by the tutor in realistic nursing interactions with the patient.
(x) On-going instruction and supervision of the student in real nursing interactions in varied and diverse nursing care contexts, by the tutor.

Intended Learning Experiences

Focus — Implementing the delivery of planned nursing care to individual patients. Using and putting nursing care plans into action as operationalised nursing care events.

Activities and Assignments in:

(i) Motivating patients and development of effective rapport.
(ii) Managing and co-ordinating the planned nursing events in varied nursing contexts.
(iii) Developing effective communication with the patient and other members of the nursing team.
(iv) Identifying, using and controlling the appropriate nursing technology (equipment and resources) to make the correct nursing interventions for individual patients.
(v) Monitoring the effects of nursing care on the patient and maintaining the nursing objectives.
(vi) Modification of objectives in relation to the specific effects of nursing care on the patient.

continued

Table 5 (continued)

Intended Instructional Events

(xi) Nursing care teaching rounds with tutor and student(s) in real clinical situations.

Intended Learning Experiences
Activities and Assignments in:

(vii) Teaching individual patients self-care within appropriate stages of the nursing care.
(viii) Using physical nursing skills to maintain the optimum physical state of the patient in varied and diverse nursing care contexts.
(ix) Coping with sudden deviations in the patient's condition and critical incidents in patient care.
(x) Dealing with accidents and emergencies and using the appropriate nursing technology and skill.

Evaluation

The identification, creation and selection of instructional events and learning experiences to develop the technical, behavioural and intellectual skills required to evaluate nursing care in varied and diverse nursing care settings.

Intended Instructional Events

Major Focus — Information processing and problem solving.

(i) Simulation exercises using assessment and evaluation procedures to determine the value and effectiveness of care given to individual patients.
(ii) Assignments of students to selected individual patients in real clinical settings to evaluate nursing care.
(iii) Tutorials, individual and group.
(iv) Tutor-led discussion groups.
(v) Student-led discussion groups.
(vi) Students using students' prepared papers on various topics of patient care evaluation.
(vii) Collaborative workshop group activities on the evaluation of selected aspects of nursing care requiring both formative and summative procedures.
(viii) Nursing care conferences with multi-disciplinary participation with the presence of selected patients or patient data to evaluate the nursing care given.
(ix) Role-play (modelling) by the tutor in making patient care evaluations in the reality of selected patient care contexts.

Intended Learning Experiences

Focus — Evaluating the effectiveness of planned individual nursing care.

Activities and Assignments in:

(i) Conceptualising evaluation and assessment and determining the differences.
(ii) Determining values and standards in nursing care.
(iii) Differentiating between qualitative and quantifiable aspects of evaluation of nursing care.
(iv) Objectivity and subjectivity in the evaluation of nursing care.
(v) Formative evaluation in varied nursing care contexts.
(vi) Summative evaluation of varied nursing care contexts.
(vii) The use of selected specific procedures of evaluation including methods of analysing, recording and synthesising data.
(viii) Acting on information and making decisions related to the outcomes of nursing care.
(ix) Observation, perception and analysis of critical incidents in nursing care.

continued

Table 5 (continued)

Intended Instructional Events	Intended Learning Experiences Activities and Assignments in:
(x) On-going instruction and supervision of the student by the tutor in varied and diverse nursing care contexts.	(x) Effecting changes in nursing care contexts using feedback during the monitoring or nursing interventions.
(xi) Using teaching rounds to evaluate nursing care contexts.	

(viii) Curriculum Evaluation and the Nursing Process

The relationship of the evaluation stage of the curriculum process, represented as phase four, is shown in alignment to the four elements of the nursing process in Figure 7. The emphasis in the evaluation of the nursing curriculum is in this study concerned with the focus of evaluation on certain aspects of the nursing process and on intended methods of evaluation which are deemed as appropriate evaluation tools. For all four phases of the nursing process the major emphasis is considered to be the student, the teacher and the use of the nursing process as an effective learning context.

Figure 7: Phase Four: The Relationship of Curriculum Evaluation to the Four Elements of the Nursing Process.

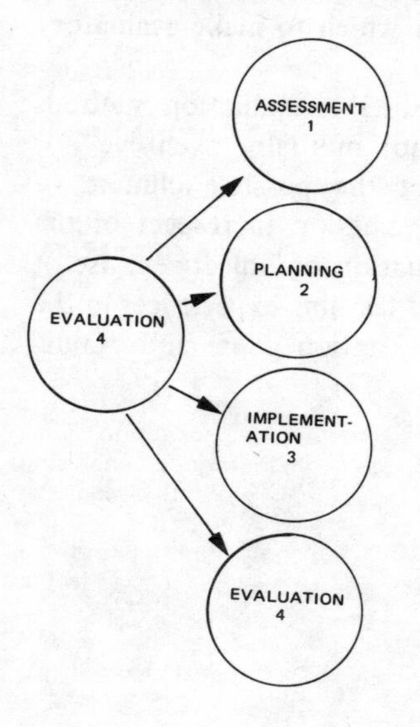

The methods of evaluation should be as comprehensive as possible using the widest range of appropriate instruments for data collecting, analysis and synthesis, including quantitative and qualitative aspects of measurement and objective and subjective aspects of evaluation. Evaluation of student achievement by teacher-made pre- and post-tests, standardised achievement tests and clinical performance tests, would be appropriate examples. The use of questionnaires and interviews, and discussions for formal and informal feedback with students, staff and teachers would be necessary. Reports from various supervising clinical nursing staff of student responses, attitudes and learning gains in various nursing care contexts regarding the use of the nursing process would be important. The teaching staff and their self-evaluations of instructional strategies used and the effectiveness of created learning experiences for students in using the nursing process would be valuable inputs to the total evaluation of the curriculum. The observations of intended and unintended results of the use of the nursing process through the evaluatory use of rating scales, check lists, systematic observation, unstructured observation and reports of involved students, clinical management staff and teachers operating in clinical settings and classrooms would be essential aspects of the evaluation. Reports, records and other data concerning recommendations and changes for improvement of the curricular arrangements for the nursing process derived from meetings and committees involving students, staff and teachers would be important sources from which to make evaluatory judgements.

The evaluation focus and examples of suitable evaluation methods are shown in Table 6. These again are not mutually exclusive nor exhaustive and simply attempt to reflect the possible climate of evaluation. The major intention of the evaluation in respect of the nursing process would be directed at evaluation of objectives, use of specific content, teaching arrangements and learning experiences in the assessment phase, planning phase, implementation phase and evaluation phase of the nursing process.

Table 6: Curriculum Evaluation and the Nursing Process

Assessment

The identification, creation and selection of evaluation procedures to estimate the value and effectiveness of the curriculum arrangements for dealing with the assessment phase of the nursing process.

Intended Methods of Evaluation
Focus — Comprehensive evaluation using a wide range of methods.

(i) Observations of intended and unintended achievement of objectives.
(ii) Achievement on teacher-made pre- and post-tests, standardised achievement tests and clinical performance tests.
(iii) Informal and formal feedback through questionnaires, interviews and discussions with students and staff.
(iv) Student observations of the influence of instruction on learning.
(v) Reports from supervising staff in the clinical settings on student responses and attitudes in nursing care interactions.
(vi) Inputs from students and tutors regarding their perceptions of the assessment phase of the nursing process.
(vii) Observation of classroom and clinical setting interactions for evidence of changes in attitude or values.
(viii) Teacher self-evaluation on instructional strategies and creation of learning experiences.
(ix) Observation of intended and unintended results of the use of the assessment phase of the nursing process, through the use of rating scales, systematic observation, unstructured observation and reports of involved students, staff and teachers.
(x) Prepare, maintain and submit reports, records and other data, and make recommendations concerning changes and improvements for curricular arrangements for the assessment phase of the nursing process.

Focus on the Evaluation of the Nursing Process Assessment Phase

(i) Student ability to identify an individual patient's nursing needs and problems.
(ii) Student ability to interview patients and take nursing histories.
(iii) Student ability to use communication techniques and knowledge of communication.
(iv) Student ability to select and use data-gathering guides and determine the correct procedures in analysis and synthesis.
(v) Student ability to make statements of cause and effect and make use of the relevant scientific facts.
(vi) Teacher instructional effectiveness and ability to create appropriate learning experiences for students in the assessment phase of the nursing process.
(vii) Quality of nursing care given to individual patients based on specific standard criteria.
(viii) The effectiveness of the assessment phase of the nursing process as an organisational tool for determining the needs and problems of the individual patient.

continued

Table 6 (continued)

Planning

The identification, creation and selection of evaluation procedures to estimate the value and effectiveness of the curriculum arrangements for dealing with the planning phase of the nursing process.

Intended Methods of Evaluation
Focus — Comprehensive evaluation using a wide range of methods.

(i) Observation of intended and unintended achievement of objectives.
(ii) Student achievement on teacher-made pre- and post-tests and clinical performance tests.
(iii) Informal and formal feedback through questionnaires, interviews and discussions with students and staff.
(iv) Reports and evidence of student observations of the influence of teacher instruction on learning.
(v) Reports from supervisory staff in the clinical settings on student abilities, responses and attitudes in nursing care interactions.
(vi) Reports from students and teachers regarding their perceptions of the planning phase of the nursing process.
(vii) Observation of classroom and clinical setting interactions for evidence of changes in attitudes or values.
(viii) Teacher self-evaluation on instructional strategies and creation of learning experiences for the planning phase of the nursing process.
(ix) Observation of intended and unintended results of the planning phase of the nursing process, through the use of rating scales, systematic observation, unstructured observation and reports of involved students, staff and teachers.
(x) Preparation, maintenance and submission of reports, records and other data, and making recommendations concerning changes and improvements for the curricular arrangements for the planning phase of the nursing process.

Focus on the Evaluation of the Planning Phase of the Nursing Process

(i) Student ability to review data systematically and define and classify problems.
(ii) Student ability to determine nursing care priorities.
(iii) Student ability to set nursing care objectives in the short, medium and long term.
(iv) Student ability to make correct and appropriate decisions related to choices in nursing care.
(v) Student ability to determine criteria for measuring the achievement of objectives.
(vi) Student ability to formulate standard (basic) nursing care plans.
(vii) Student ability to formulate individual (unique) nursing care plans.
(viii) Student ability to consult, collaborate and communicate in the formulation of nursing care plans.
(ix) Teacher instructional effectiveness and ability to create appropriate learning experiences for students in the planning stage of the nursing process.
(x) Quality of intended nursing care based on specific standard criteria.
(xi) The effectiveness of the planning phase of the nursing process as an organisational tool for determining the nature and form of nursing care to be given.

continued

Table 6 (continued)

Implementation

The identification, creation and selection of evaluation procedures to estimate the value and effectiveness of the curriculum arrangements for dealing with the implementation phase of the nursing process.

Intended Methods of Evaluation	Focus on the Evaluation of the Implementation phase of the Nursing Process
Focus – Comprehensive evaluation using a wide range of methods.	
(i) Observation of intended and unintended achievement of objectives.	(i) Student ability to motivate patients.
(ii) Student achievement on teacher-made pre- and post-tests, standardised achievement tests and clinical performance tests.	(ii) Student ability to manage and co-ordinate planned nursing events.
(iii) Informal and formal feedback through questionnaires, interviews and discussions with students and staff.	(iii) Student ability to communicate during the implementation of nursing care.
(iv) Reports and evidence of student observations of the influence of teacher instruction on learning.	(iv) Student ability to select, use and control appropriate resources and nursing technology during the implementation of individual nursing care in varied nursing contexts.
(v) Reports from supervising staff in the clinical settings on student abilities, responses and attitudes in nursing care interactions.	(v) Student ability to monitor nursing care and maintain the intentions of the planned care.
(vi) Reports from students and teachers regarding their perceptions of the implementation phase of the nursing process.	(vi) Student ability to respond to changes and modify nursing objectives.
(vii) Observation of classroom and clinical setting interactions for evidence of changes in attitudes or values.	(vii) Student ability to teach the patient self-care as appropriate.
(viii) Teacher self-evaluation of instructional strategies and creation of learning experiences for the implementation phase of the nursing process.	(viii) Student ability to use nursing skills to maintain the optimum physical state of the patient in varied and diverse nursing care contexts.
(ix) Observation of intended and unintended results of the implementation phase of the nursing process, through the use of rating scales, systematic observation, unstructured observation and reports of involved students, staff and teachers.	(ix) Student ability to deal with specific critical incidents in nursing care.
(x) Preparation, maintenance and supervision of reports, records and other data, and making recommendations concerning changes and improvements for the curricular	(x) Student ability to deal with accidents and emergency events, using the appropriate nursing technology and skills.
	(xi) Teacher instructional effectiveness and ability to create appropriate learning experiences for students in the implementation phase of the nursing process.
	(xii) Quality of nursing care during implementation phase of the nursing process based on specific standard criteria.

continued

Table 6 (continued)

arrangements for the implementation phase of the nursing process.	(xiii) The effectiveness of the implementation phase of the nursing process as a tool for organising the delivery of care to the patient.

Evaluation

The identification, creation and selection of evaluation procedures to estimate the value and effectiveness of the curriculum arrangements for dealing with the evaluation phase of the nursing process.

Intended Methods of Evaluation	**Focus on the Evaluation of the Evaluation Phase of the Nursing Process**
Focus — Comprehensive evaluation using a wide range of methods.	
(i) Observation of intended and unintended achievement of objectives.	(i) Student ability to conceptualise evaluation and assessment and determine differences.
(ii) Student achievement on teacher-made pre- and post-tests, standardised achievement tests and clinical performance tests.	(ii) Student ability to determine and use values and standards in nursing care events.
(iii) Informal and formal feedback through questionnaires, interviews and discussions with students and staff.	(iii) Student ability to make qualitative and quantifiable evaluations of nursing care.
(iv) Reports and evidence of student observations of the influence of teacher instruction on learning.	(iv) Student ability to make objective and subjective evaluations of nursing care.
(v) Reports from supervising staff in the clinical settings on student abilities, responses and attitudes in nursing care interactions.	(v) Student ability to make formative and summative evaluations in varied and diverse nursing care contexts.
(vi) Reports from students and teachers regarding their perceptions of the implementation phase of the nursing process.	(vi) Student ability to select and use appropriate evaluation procedures.
(vii) Observation of classroom and clinical setting interactions for evidence of changes in attitudes or values.	(vii) Student ability in perception, observation and analysis of critical nursing incidents.
(viii) Teacher self-evaluation on instructional strategies and the creation of learning experiences for the evaluation phase of the nursing process.	(viii) Student ability to make use of feedback to effect changes in the form, nature and quality of nursing care.
(ix) Observation of intended and unintended results of the evaluation phase of the nursing process, through the use of rating scales, systematic observation, unstructured observation and reports of involved students, staff and teachers.	(ix) Teacher effectiveness in instructional contexts and ability to create effective learning experiences for students in the evaluation phase of the nursing process.
	(x) Quality of nursing care during the evaluation phase of the nursing process resulting from specific evaluative procedures and outcomes.

continued

Table 6 (continued)

(x) Preparation, maintenance and submission of reports, records and other data, and making recommendations concerning improvements and changes for the curricular arrangements for the evaluation phase of the nursing process.	(xi) The effectiveness of the evaluation phase of the nursing process as a tool for improving individual nursing care.

(ix) Conclusion

In this final chapter an attempt has been made to suggest, by using a curriculum process, certain objectives, content, learning activities and evaluation procedures, and an adaptation of the nursing process as a series of themes or organising centres to provide a suitable framework for the nursing curriculum. In this way a nursing curriculum model has been proposed which can be used to reach decisions and facilitate effective curricular plans for using the antecedent and specific knowledge of nursing.

In using the model it is important to view it as an educational model which uses the nursing process to enable students to learn fundamental principles, concepts and facts about an individual patient's problems and the application of nursing interventions to reduce these problems by objective, planned and evaluated nursing care. In this educational context the nursing process must also be seen to serve as an educational instrument by which students can consistently follow the steps of the problem-solving process, so that they can learn about nursing in terms of its functional nature, its interventions, its roles and its technologies.

The nursing curriculum model must prepare the students for the intellectual, technical and behavioural process required for designing, delivering, controlling and evaluating organised nursing care. The principles that students learn, the nursing abilities that they develop, apply and evaluate, and the general spectrum of problems they identify and analyse should result in an educational experience in nursing care that prepares them to be competent, accountable professional nurses. The proposed model seeks to plan and develop these experiences for students of modern professional nursing.

Most models are conceptual representations of reality – not reality itself, but an abstracted reconstruction of it. This means that all models have their limitations, and turning abstract concepts into practice is a difficult business. Nevertheless a conceptual model for the curriculum can provide a necessary working structure for thinking about the way in which a course, programme or educational system might work.

It would seem that whether a school of nursing uses a particular nursing model or not, four major aspects of the curriculum are influenced by the nursing process construct of nursing care. These four major aspects are the intended objectives of the courses, the selected content of the courses, the methods used to teach and learn the content, and the development of procedures to evaluate the courses. These four curricular elements are the essential structural fabric and functional processes of the operational curriculum.

The nursing process, with its concern for objective approaches, planned care and effective evaluation procedures, has strikingly similar form and mode to the curriculum process. The nature of thinking required for both is similar in that it is logical, systematic and has major practical application directed at particular ends. Although these ends are different, there exists considerable similarity. The ends in the nursing process are concerned with effective care of the patient and the process itself provides the means by which the ends are achieved. The ends in the curriculum process are concerned with the production of effective nurses to care for the patient and the process itself provides the educational means by which such ends are achieved.

Nurse educators should be concerned with the means and the ends in both the nursing of patients and the education of nurses to be effective practitioners.

It is with both means and ends in mind, with regard to nursing practice and nursing education, that this model has been offered and it is hoped that in a modest way it may provide guidance for those who seek to educate nurses.

BIBLIOGRAPHY

Abdellah, F.G. (1965). The nature of nursing science. *Nursing Research, 18,* 390-3

Abdellah, F.G., Beland, I., Martin, A. and Matheney, R. (1960). *New Directions in Patient Centred Nursing,* New York, Collier-Macmillan.

Alpern, D.K. (1966). In place of recitations: an experiment in teaching. *Teachers College Records, 67,* 589-94.

Altschul, A.T. (1978). A systems approach to the nursing process. *Journal of Advanced Nursing, 3, 4,* 333-40.

Anderson, O.R. (1971). *The Quantitative Analysis of Structure in Teaching,* New York Teachers College Press.

Anderson, N.E. (1981). The historical development of American nursing education. *Journal of Nursing Education, 20* (1 January) 18-35.

Anderson, R.C. (1967). Educational psychology. *Annual Review of Psychology, 18,* 129-64.

Armstrong-Esther, E. (1979). Address given at the Annual Conference of the Association of Health Careers Advisors, April 1979, reported in *Nursing Times* (26 April), 695.

Atkins, J.M. (1968). Behavioural objectives in curriculum design: a cautionary note. *The Science Teacher* (May), 27-30.

Ausubel, D.P. (1967). *Learning Theory and Classroom Practice,* Toronto, Ontario, Institute of Studies in Education.

Baker, G.L. and Goldberg, I. (1970). Individualized learning system: what it is and how to use it. *Educational Leadership, 27,* (8 May), 775-80.

Batey, V. (1977). Conceptualisation: knowledge and logic guiding and empirical research. *Nursing Research, 26, 54* (Sept/Oct), 324-9.

Beattie, A. (1979). A structural map of health care models (Unpublished seminar notes).

Bernstein, B. (1971). On the classification and framing of educational knowledge. In (M. Young, ed.) *Knowledge and Control,* London, Collier Macmillan.

Bloom, B.S. (1956). *Taxonomy of Educational Objectives, Volume 1, Cognitive Domain,* New York, McKay.

—— (1958). Ideas, problems, and methods of inquiry. In *The Integration of Educational Experience.* Fifty Seventh Year Book of the National Society for the Study of Education, Part III, University of Chicago Press, pp. 84-104.

—— (1976). *Human Characteristics and School Learning,* New York, McGraw-Hill.

Bobbit, J.F. (1924). *How to Make a Curriculum,* Boston, Houghton Mifflin.

Boe, G.P. (1980). A systems approach to curriculum evaluation in vocational-technical education. *Journal of American Medical Technology, 42,* 17-19.

Bolvin, J.O. (1968). Implications of the individualization of instruction for curriculum and instructional design. *Audiovisual Instruction, 13, 3* (March), 238-42.

Briggs, L.J. (1967). *Sequencing of Instruction in Relation to Hierarchies of Competence,* Chicago, American Institute for Research, Monograph No. 3.

Brodbeck, M. (1969). Models, meanings and theories. In (M. Brodbeck, ed.) *Readings in the Philosophy of Social Sciences,* London, Collier-Macmillan.

Brown, S.J. (1980). The nursing process systems model. *Journal of Nursing Education, 20, 6* (June), 36-40.

Bruner, J.S. (1960). *The Process of Education*, New York, Vintage Books, Random House.
—— (1971). *The Process of Education*, New York, Norton.
Bush, H.A. (1979). Models for nursing. *Advances in Nursing Science, 1* (January), 13-21.
Carol, J.B. (1963). A model of school learning. *Teachers College Record, 64*, 723-33.
Charters, W.W. and Waples, D. (1929). *The Commonwealth Teacher Training Study*, Chicago, University of Chicago Press.
Chater, S.S. (1975). A conceptual framework for curriculum development. *Nursing Outlook, 23, 7*, 428-33.
Collins, S.M. (1981). Nursing the next 100 years. *Journal of Advanced Nursing, 6, 3*, 165-71.
Corona, D. (1979). A continuous progress curriculum in nursing. *Nursing Outlook* (January), 46-8.
Christman, M. and Riehl, J. (1974). Developmental models. The systems development stress model. In (J.R. Riehl and C. Roy, eds), *Conceptual Models for Nursing Practice*, New York, Appleton-Century-Crofts, pp. 247-68.
Cronhach, L.J. (1967). How can instruction be adapted to individual differences? In (R.M. Gagné, ed.), *Learning and Individual Differences*, Columbus, Ohio, Merrill, pp. 22-9.
Crow, R. (1981). Speculation on the concept of nursing. Address given at the International Council of Nursing 17th Quadrennial Congress, Los Angeles, California. Reported in *Nursing Standard, 203* (23 July).
Curtin, L. (1979). The nurse as advocate: a philosophical foundation for nursing. *Advances in Nursing Science, 1, 3*.
Davies, I.K. (1976) *Objectives in Curriculum Design*, New York, McGraw-Hill.
Derdiarian, A.K. (1979). Education: a way to theory construction in nursing. *Journal of Nursing Education, 18, 2*, 36-47.
Dickoff, J. and James, P. (1968). A theory of theories: a position paper. *Nursing Research, 17*, 415-35.
—— (1970). Beliefs and values: bases for curriculum design. *Nursing Research, 19*, 415-27.
Dirkzwager, A. (1974). Computer-based testing with automatic scoring of subjective probabilities. Paper given at the 2nd World Congress of IFIP on Computers in Education, Marseilles.
Duffey, M. and Mullenkamp, A.F. (1974). A framework for theory analysis. *Nursing Outlook, 22*, 570-4.
Dyer, M. (1979). *The Process of Change and the Curriculum Design in Designing and Building a Curriculum*, National League for Nursing, New York, Pub. No. 16. 1776.
Eisner, E.W. (1979). *The Educational Imagination: On the Design and Evaluation of School Programmes*, New York, Macmillan.
Ellis, R. (1973). Characteristics of significant theories. In (M.E. Hardy, ed.) *Theoretical Foundations for Nursing*, New York, MSS Information Corporation.
Elshout, R. and Elshout, M. (1969). The programmed instruction of problem solving. In (F. Besson and D. de Montmollin, eds) *Programmed Learning Research*, Paris, Dunod.
Erickson, E. (1959). *Identity and the Life Cycle.* Psychological Issues, Monograph, Vol. 1, New York, International Universities Press.
Finch, C.R. and Bjorkquist, D.C. (1977). Review and critique of context and input measures in evaluation. Journal of Industrial Teacher Education, *14, 2*, 7-18.

Flint, J.W. (1980). The nursing systems analyst: are you ready for her? *Supervision Nurse, 11* (January), 55-6.
Frase, L.T. (1975). Advances in research and theory in instructional technology. In (F.N. Kerlinger, ed.) *Review of Research in Education, Vol. 3*, Itascia, Illinois, Peacock.
Freud, S. (1922). *Group Psychology and the Analysis of the Ego*, New York, International Psychoanalytical Press.
Fuller, F.F. (1969). Concerns of teachers: a developmental conceptualisation. *American Educational Research Journal, 6*, 207-26.
Gagné, R.M. (1965). *The Conditions of Learning*, New York, Holt, Rinehart and Winston Inc.
Gagné, R.M. and Briggs, L.J. (1974). *Principles of Instructional Design*, New York, Holt, Rinehart and Winston Inc.
Gagné, R.M. and Rowher, W.D. Jr. (1969). Instructional psychology. *Annual Review of Psychology, 20*, 351-418.
Gagné, R.M. and White, R.T. (1978) Memory structures and learning outcomes. *Review of Educational Research, 48*, 187-222.
Glaser, R. (1963). Instructional technology and the measurement of learning outcomes. *American Psychologist, 18*, 519-21.
—— (1967). Psychology and instructional technology. In (R. Glaser, ed) *Training Research and Education*, Pittsburgh, University of Pittsburgh Press.
Glaser, R. and Resnick, K.B. (1970). Instructional psychology. *Annual Review of Psychology, 23*, 207-76.
Goodland, J.I. and Richter, M.N. Jr. (1963). The development of a conceptual system for dealing with problems of curriculum and instruction. USOE Contract No. SAE8024, Project No. 454, University of California, Los Angeles.
Greaves, F. (1980). Objectively towards curriculum development in nursing education in England and Wales. *Journal of Advanced Nursing, 5*, 591-9.
—— (1982). Innovation, change, decision making and the key variables in nursing curriculum implementation. *International Journal of Nursing Studies, 19, 1*, 11-19.
Griggs, B.M. (1977). A systems approach to the development and evaluation of a mini course for nurses. *Nursing Research, 26, 1*, 34-41.
Hamilton, R.H. (1967). An experiment with independent study in freshman history. *Liberal Education, 53*, 271-8.
Hardy, M.E. (1973). The nature of theories. In (M.E. Hardy, ed.) *Theoretical Foundations for Nursing*, New York MSS Information Corporation.
Harmer, B. (1922). *Textbook of the Principles and Practice of Nursing*, New York, Macmillan.
Harms, M.J. and McDonald, F.G. (1966). A new curriculum design. *Nursing Outlook* (September), 50-3.
Harrow, A.J. (1972). *A Taxonomy of the Psycho-Motor Domain*, New York, McKay.
Heidergerken, L. (1955). When is a course integrated? *Nursing Outlook, 3* (March), 128-9.
Henderson, V. (1966). *The Nature of Nursing*, New York, Macmillan.
—— (1978). The concept of nursing. *Journal of Advanced Nursing, 3, 2* 113-30.
Henry, N.B. (1958). *The Integration of Educational Experiences*. The Fifty Seventh Year Book of the National Society for the Study of Education, Part III, Chicago, University of Chicago Press, p. 11.
Herrick, V.E. and Tyler, R.W. (1950) *Toward Improved Curriculum Theory*, Supplementary Educational Monograph, No. 71, Chicago, University of Chicago Press.

Hide, S.E. (1981). Teaching the ethical component of nursing. *Nurse Education Today, 1, 2,* 22-4.
Hipps, O.S. (1981). The integrated curriculum: the Emperor is naked. *American Journal of Nursing, 81, 5,* 976-80.
Hirst, P.H. (1968). The logical and psychological aspects of teaching a subject. In (R.D. Peters, ed.) *The Concept of Education*, London Routledge and Kegan Paul, p. 45.
—— (1975). Curriculum objectives. In (P.H. Hirst) *Knowledge and the Curriculum*, London, Routledge and Kegan Paul.
Hooper, R. (ed.) (1971). *The Curriculum: Context, Design and Development*, Edinburgh, Oliver and Boyd, pp. 117-23.
Hopkins, L.T. (1935). Arguments for favouring integration. *Teachers College Record, 36*, 604-12.
Jaffee, M. *et al.* (1979). Specialist in an integrated curriculum: an odyssey. *Journal of Nursing Education, 18*, 46-9.
Johansen, D. (1951). Integration-correlation. *American Journal of Nursing, 51*, 405-6.
Johnson, D.E. (1968a). One conceptual model of nursing. Paper presented at Vanderbilt University, Nashville, Tennessee, 25 April.
—— (1968b). Theory in nursing: borrowed and unique. *Nursing Research, 17*, 206-9.
Johnson, M. (1967). Definitions and models in curriculum theory. *Educational Theory, 17*, 127-40.
Keller, F.S. (1978). Goodbye teacher. In (J. Hartley and J.K. Davies, eds) *Contributions to an Educational Technology, Vol. II*, London, Kogan Page.
Kemp, J.E. (1971). *Instructional Design*, Palo Alto, California, Fearon Publishers.
Kerr, J. (1968). *Changing the Curriculum*, London, University of London Press.
Ketefian, S. (1978). Strategies of curriculum change. *International Nursing Review, 25, 1*, 14-21.
King, I.M. (1968). A conceptual framework of reference for nursing. *Nursing Research, 17*, 27-31.
—— (1970). *Toward a Theory for Nursing*, New York, John Wiley & Sons.
—— (1975). A process for developing coneepts for nursing through research. In (P.J. Veronick, ed) *Nursing Research, Vol. 1*, Boston, Little, Brown & Co.
Klix, S. (1971). Information unt verhalpen, kybernetische aspekta der organismischen information verar beitung-econfuhrung. In *Naturwissenschaftliche Grundlagen der allgemeinen Psychologie*, Berlin, Deutscher Verlag der Wissenschaften.
Kneller, G.F. (1972). Behavioural objectives? No! *Educational Leadership, 29, 5*, 397-400.
Knudsen, C.W. (1937). What do educators mean by 'integration'? *Harvard Educational Review, 12*, 15-26.
Krathwohl, D.R., Bloom, B.S. and Masia, B.B. (1964). *Taxonomy of Educational Objectives. Handbook II: The Affective Domain*, New York, McKay.
Leininger, M. (1978). *Transcultural Nursing: Concepts, Theories, and Practices*, New York, John Wiley.
Levine, L.B. (1979). Through the looking class at the integrated curriculum. *Journal of Nursing Education, 18, 7*, 43-6.
MacDonald-Ross, M. (1973). Behavioural objectives: a critical review. *Instructional Science, 2*, 1-52.

Mager, R. (1967). *Preparing Instructional Objectives*, Palo Alto, California, Fearon.

Maslow, A.H. (1970). *Motivation and Personality*, 2nd edn, New York, Harper & Row.

Mayers, M.G. (1978). *A Systems Approach to the Nursing Care Plan*, 2nd edn, New York, Appleton-Century-Crofts.

McCarthy, M.M. (1981). The nursing process: application of current thinking in clinical problem solving. *Journal of Advanced Nursing, 6, 3*, 173-7.

McCloskey, J.C. (1981). The professionalisation of nursing: United States and England. *International Nursing Review, 28, 2*, 40-7.

McFarlane, E.A. (1980). Nursing theory: the comparison of four theoretical proposals. *Journal of Advanced Nursing, 5*, 3-19.

McFarlane, J.K. (1977). Developing a theory of nursing: the relation of theory to practice, education and research. *Journal of Advanced Nursing, 2*, 261-70.

McKay, R. (1973). Theories, models and systems for nursing. In (M.E. Hardy, ed.) *Theoretical Foundations for Nursing*, New York, MSS Information Corporation.

McKeachie, W.J. (1974). Instructional psychology. *Annual Review of Psychology, 25*, 161-93.

Meleis, A.I. (1979). The Development of a conceptually based nursing curriculum: an international experiment. *Journal of Advanced Nursing, 4*, 659-71.

Miller, M. (1980). The revised curriculum. *Journal of Emergency Nursing, 6* (Jan./Feb.), 42-3.

Mitchell, P.H. (1977). *Concepts Basic to Nursing*, New York, McGraw-Hill.

Moritz, D.A. (1979). Primary nursing: implications for curriculum development. *Journal of Nursing Education, 18, 3*, 32-7.

National League for Nursing (1974). *Faculty Curriculum Development*, New York, The National League for Nursing.

Neuman, M. (1972). Nursing's theoretical evolution. *Nursing Outlook, 20*, 449-53.

Newman, B. and Young, R.J. (1972). A model for teaching a total person approach to patient problems. *Nursing Research, 21, 3*

Norton, D. (1981). The quiet revolution: introduction of the nursing process in a region. *Nursing Times, 77, 25* (17-23 June), 1067-9.

Notter, L.E. and Robey, M. (1979). The open curriculum in nursing education. Final Report of the National League for Nursing Open Curriculum Study, Pub. No. 19, New York.

Novello, D.J. (1976). Proliferating curriculums. In J.A. Williamson, ed.) *Current Perspectives in Nursing Education. The Changing Scene*, St Louis, C.V. Mosby, pp. 66-73.

Olsen, V. (1979). Overcoming crises in a new nursing programme. Mt Hood Community College. In (G. Grant, ed.) *On Competence. A Critical Analysis of Competence-based Reforms in Higher Education*, San Francisco, Josey Bass, pp. 335-62.

Orem, D.E. (1971). *Nursing: Concepts of Practice*, New York, McGraw-Hill.

Orlando, I.J. (1961). *The Dynamic Nurse-Patient Relationship*, New York, G.P. Putnams & Sons.

Parker, F.W. (1894). *Talks on Pedagogics: the Outline of the Theory of Concentration*, New York, Kellog.

Parsons, M.A. (1980). The process of change in curriculum evaluation. *Journal of Nursing Education, 19, 7*, 36-8.

Paterson, J.G. and Zderad, L.T. (1976). *Humanistic Nursing*, New York, John Wiley & Sons.

Peterson, C.J. (1977). Questions frequently asked about the development of conceptual framework. *Journal of Nursing Education, 16, 4*, 22-32.

Phenix, P.H. (1964). *Realms of Meaning*, New York, McGraw-Hill.

Pletsch, P.K. (1979). Intrapartum practicum in nursing curricula. *Journal of Nursing Education, 18, 9*, 26-9.

Popham, J. (1969). *Instructional Objectives*, Palo Alto, California, Fearon.

Postner, G.J. (1974). The extensiveness of curriculum structure: a conceptual scheme. *Review of Educational Research, 44, 4*, 401-6.

Quinn, F.M. (1980). *The Principles and Practice of Nurse Education*, London, Croom Helm.

Reilly, D.E. (1975). Why a conceptual framework? *Nursing Outlook, 23*, 566-9.

Rogers, C.R. (1951). *Client Centered Therapy*, Boston, Houghton Mifflin & Co.

Rogers, M.E. (1970). *An Introduction to the Theoretical Basis of Nursing*, Philadelphia, F.A. Davis.

Roper, N. (1976). *Clinical Experience in Nurse Education*, University of Edinburgh, Department of Nursing Studies, Monograph No. 5, Edinburgh Churchill Livingstone.

Roy, S.C. (1970). Adaptation: a conceptual framework for nursing. *Nursing Outlook, 18*, 42-5.

—— (1971). Adaptation: a basis for nursing practice. *Nursing Outlook, 19*, 254-7.

—— (1976). *Introduction to Nursing: An Adaptation Model*, Englewood Cliffs, New Jersey, Prentice-Hall.

Scholtfeldt, T. (1972). The need for a conceptual framework. In (P.J. Verhonick, ed) *Nursing Research, Vol. 1*, Boston, Little, Brown & Co.

Schrader, B.H. (1972). Function and group as unifying themes in secondary school algebra. Unpublished doctoral dissertation, State University of New York at Albany.

Schwab, J.J. (1969). The practical: a language for curriculum. *School Review, 78*, 1-23.

Scriven, M. (1967): The methodology of evaluation. In (B. Worthen and J. Sanders, eds) *Educational Evaluation: Theory and Practice*, Charles A. Jones, Worthington, Ohio, pp. 60-104.

Sculco, C.D. (1978). Development of a taxonomy for the nursing process. *Journal of Nursing Education, 17*, 40-8.

Shaw, C.S.W. (1902). *A Textbook for Nursing*, 3rd edn, New York, Appleton-Century-Crofts.

Sheahan, J. (1980). Some aspects of the teaching and learning of nursing. *Journal of Advanced Nursing, 5*, 491-511.

Shufflebeam, D.Z. (1969). *Evaluation as Enlightenment for Decision-Making. Improving Educational Assessment*, Washington, D.C., Association for Supervision and Curriculum Development, National Education Association.

Simms, L.L. (1973). Impact of patient centred approaches on the emergency role of the clinical nurse specialist. In (F.G. Abdellah, Beland, I., Martin, A. and Matheney, R., eds) *New Directions in Patient Centred Nursing*, 2nd edn, New York, Collier-Macmillan, p. 95

Smeltzer, C. (1980). Teaching the nursing process – practical method. *Journal of Nursing Education, 19, 9*, 31-7.

Stenhouse, L. (1970). Some limitations of the use of objectives in curriculum research and planning. *Pedagogica Europea*, 75-83.

Styles, M.M. (1976). In the name of integration. *Nursing Outlook, 24*, 738-44.
Sullivan, T.J. (1977). An experience with a systems approach to curriculum design. *Journal of Nursing Education, 16, 3*, 25-33.
Taba, H. (1962). *Curriculum Development Theory and Practice*, New York, Harcourt Brace.
Torres, G. (1974). Educational trends and the integrated curriculum approach in nursing. In *Faculty Curriculum Development, Part IV. Unifying the Curriculum – The Integrated Approach*, New York, National League for Nursing, pp. 1-6.
Torres, G. and Yura, H. (1974). *Today's Conceptual Framework, its Relationship to Curriculum Process*, New York, National League for Nursing, Pub. No. 15. 1529.
Treffinger, D.G. (1977). *Handbook on Teaching Educational Psychology*, New York and London, Academic Press.
Tyler, R.W. (1950). *The Basic Principles of Curriculum and Instruction*, Chicago, University of Chicago Press.
Weitzel, M.H. (1980). Philosophical base for the integrated nursing curriculum. *Nursing Leadership, 18, 3*, 17-37.
Welch, L.B. and Slagle, J.C. (1980). Does integrated content lead to integrated curriculum? *Journal of Nursing Education, 19*, 38-40.
Wentling, T.L. and Lawson, T.E. (1975). *Evaluating Occupational Education and Training Programmes*, Boston, Allyn and Bacon Inc.
Wheeler, D.K. (1967). *Curriculum Process*, London, Unibooks, University of London Press.
Whelton, B.J. (1979). An operationalization of Martha Roger's theory throughout the nursing process. *International Journal of Nursing Studies, 16*, 7-20.
Wiedenbach, E. (1964). *Clinical Nursing: A Helping Art*, New York, Springer Publishing Co.
Williamson, J.A. (ed.) (1976). *Current Perspectives in Nursing Education*. The Changing Scene. St Louis, C.V. Mosby.
Wu, R.R. (1979). Designing a curriculum model. *Journal of Nursing Education, 18, 3*, 13-21.

Reports and Acts

General Nursing Council (1981). *A New Syllabus for Mental Nursing*. Consultative Document.
General Nursing Council (1981). *A New Syllabus for the Mentally Subnormal*. Consultative Document.
National League of Nursing (1917). *Curriculum Committee*, National League of Nursing, New York.
—— (1927). *A Standard Curriculum for Schools of Nursing*, National League of Nursing, New York.
—— (1937). *A Curriculum Guide for Schools of Nursing*, Committee on Curriculum of the National League of Nursing, New York.
Nurses, Health Visitors and Midwives Act, 1979.
Report of the Committee on Nursing. Chairman, Asa Briggs. Cmnd 5115, London, HMSO, 1972.

INDEX